It's Not Your Fault!

IT'S NOT YOUR FAULT!

Strategies for Solving Toilet Training and Bedwetting Problems

JOSEPH BARONE, MD

RUTGERS UNIVERSITY PRESS
New Brunswick, New Jersey, and London

Library of Congress Cataloging-in-Publication Data
Barone, Joseph, 1959–
    It's not your fault! : strategies for solving toilet training and bedwetting
problems / Joseph Barone, MD.
        pages cm
    Includes bibliographical references and index.
    ISBN 978–0–8135–6992–5 (paperback) — ISBN 978–0–8135–6993–2
(e-book)
    1. Toilet training. 2. Enuresis. I. Title.
    HQ770.5.B37 2015
    649'62—dc23   2014017495

A British Cataloging-in-Publication record for this book is available from the
    British Library.

Visit our website: http://rutgerspress.rutgers.edu

Manufactured in the United States of America

CONTENTS

INTRODUCTION

It's not your fault! That is what I tell frustrated parents who visit me because they are not able to toilet train their child. In most of these cases, the parents followed well-meaning but generally bad advice they discovered in a parenting book, on the Internet, or during a popular TV talk show.

Once, a mother of a thirteen-month-old told me that her friend, who regularly beat her at tennis, trained her perfect eleven-month-old by holding the baby over the toilet until blastoff. When the losing tennis player tried that method with her thirteen-month-old, she was crushed because that method did not work for her. She felt like she did something wrong and somehow failed her child and lost to her tennis friend yet again. Of course, I told her, "It's not your fault." After all, she did not do anything wrong, she was just given well-meaning but bad advice from her friend. This advice may work well for one person but not for another.

In this book, I want to provide evidence-based advice and share my twenty-year experience as a pediatric urologist. "Evidence-based advice" means that the advice is based on science and facts. It means that it is more than just someone's personal opinion—it is advice based on testing and research. Evidence-based advice is the best advice available, and you should demand the best advice for your child. When advice is evidence based, it should work for many people, not just for one person, as in the tennis player example.

I am not only a pediatric urologist; I am also a father of four with a perfect toilet training batting average, and that did not happen by "accident." I know my recommendations for toilet training work because they have been tested and have proven to be effective in the real world, as well as in a research setting. In fact, for the last ten years, I have spent thousands of hours gathering the large amount of information that is contained in this book. I want to pass that information on to you. And because my recommendations are evidence based, they work for everyone, not just that one tennis player.

The reason a lot of information on toilet training is misleading (or just plain wrong) is because very few scientific studies have been performed to help us better understand toilet training. Did you know that there are thousands of scientific studies on asthma but less than a few dozen studies on toilet training? With that kind of knowledge gap, we should not be surprised that, each year, over seven million children develop some kind of toilet training problem, like delayed toilet training, day wetting, or bedwetting. All of these common problems are discussed here, and following the toilet training advice in this book will prevent many of these problems from occurring in your child. In many cases, these problems could have been prevented if parents had access to evidence-based toilet training information instead of someone's personal opinion.

Even though toilet training is a natural process, understanding some simple but important facts will allow parents to successfully and quickly train their children and avoid mountains of problems and years of disappointment. I am excited to share the information contained in this book because it has resulted from a lifetime of work, study, experience, and fun. The message I want to get across is that all parents can successfully and quickly toilet train their children, provided they have the essential, evidence-based information I provide here. And, if things do not go according to plan and a potty training problem occurs, you are covered: this book will tell you how to deal with common potty training problems like bedwetting or daytime wetting.

ABOUT ME

I would like to tell you a little bit about my training and experience so you can understand where—literally—I'm coming from. I am chief of pediatric urology at Rutgers–Robert Wood Johnson Medical School, located in New Brunswick, New Jersey. This position allows me to research urinary control problems in children and to find and develop new ways to think about these problems. I am like a detective trying to solve a mystery. I am also surgeon-in-chief at the Bristol-Myers Squibb Children's Hospital at Robert Wood Johnson University Hospital, also located in New Brunswick. It is there that my colleagues and I have our pediatric continence center and where we have treated thousands of children with urinary control issues, from the most common to the most complex.

I think that a person's background and experience can really influence how he views things, and they affect the way he responds to different situations. Understanding a little bit about me personally might therefore help you understand how I have developed the concepts and recommendations that are contained in this book. I also want you to be able to see me as a person, not only as a professional writing a textbook. I would like to connect to you on a personal level because the main purpose of this book is to help you properly toilet train your child and also to help you overcome any toilet training problems your child might have or develop in the future. I want you to feel confident and comfortable with my recommendations so you can take charge of the situation and make things better for you and your child.

As I mentioned in the introduction, I have real-life experience in toilet training as a father and husband. My wife Anne Marie and I have successfully toilet trained our children following the simple principles outlined in this book. I admit that we are at somewhat of an advantage since I am a pediatric urologist and Anne Marie is a registered nurse, but the purpose of this book is to transfer that knowledge to you so that you can be equally successful in your home with your family.

I am fully trained and board certified in adult urology and pediatric urology. But I practice only pediatric urology, and almost 40 percent of my practice has to do with the management of children with different types of potty training and urinary control issues. These potty training issues might include problems like delayed toilet training, daytime urinary wetting, and bedwetting. This means that I have treated thousands of children with all kinds of urinary control issues over the years. There is virtually no problem that I have not seen and treated. I will address the more common of these problems in this book, and I will provide you with the same information and detailed advice that I provide to parents who come to my office for a formal consultation.

For the last fifteen years, I have also been medical director of the Pediatric Continence Center at the Bristol-Myers Squibb Children's Hospital at Robert Wood Johnson University Hospital. I developed this center fifteen years ago because I saw a need to have a place where common toilet training problems and questions could be studied and treated. Toilet training problems are very common, even if they are not talked about that much. Let's face it, talking about your child's potty training problem does not make for the best teatime conversation. The Pediatric Continence Center provides a place where these very common problems can be openly discussed and addressed.

Our Pediatric Continence Center is now a major referral center for children with all kinds of urinary control problems, and we have specialized equipment and testing abilities at the center to examine children in more detail when necessary. You will learn about these tests later in the book, but I hope you will never need our services. The nursing director at the center who helps me care for our patients is Eileen Creenan. Eileen is a pediatric urology nurse with decades of experience treating children with different types of urinary control problems. We will hear more from Eileen later on this book, where I interview her and get a nursing perspective on common toilet training problems. She has managed thousands of children with me over the last fifteen years.

In addition to my experience as a pediatric urologist and clinician, I have written hundreds of scientific papers and done research on toilet training, daytime wetting, and nighttime urinary control problems in children. This is the evidence-based information that I mentioned in the introduction, and I often refer to it throughout this book. Some of my research provides the only evidence-based information available to help us understand toilet training and urinary control problems in children. It is truly valuable information because it is based, not on opinion, but on facts.

I started to do research in this area because there was a real need for good, solid evidence-based information on this topic. Even though toilet training is an important topic and a major milestone in child development, there have been very few studies done to understand how a child gains urinary control and what to do when things go wrong. I wanted to fix that situation by studying this topic and writing about my findings in this book. The research that I have done in the past has been evaluated and published in prestigious scientific journals. I would like to present that information to you using language that is understandable to moms and dads who may not be medically trained, parents who wish to properly toilet train their child or who want to help their child overcome a toilet training problem. I would like you to trust the evidence-based information that is presented in this book because it is backed by high-quality research and is not just a statement of personal opinion.

Because I have treated so many families whose children have different types of potty training issues, I understand how difficult these problems can be. I understand that hearing someone say that your child will "outgrow" a potty training problem can be frustrating. I know that most children and parents want these problems to go away as soon as possible and don't want to wait years and years for the child to "outgrow" the problem. I have also seen parents become frustrated simply because there was no place to turn for good solid evidence-based advice or reliable information.

I have seen thousands of potty training problems cause difficulties for families, problems ranging from teasing between siblings to arguments between parents that have led to divorce. Yes, it can get that frustrating. Understandably, parents can grow apprehensive when their child cannot toilet train, and they may start to blame the child, themselves, or each other for the problems they are experiencing. These types of feelings are not abnormal, but they are not appropriate, either. It's not your fault, but it's not your child's or spouse's fault, either. I hope that by reading this book you will be able to successfully toilet train your child and to also better understand why your child might be having a potty training problem. The information that is contained in this book will put you in a better position to help your child potty train; it's that simple. As you read this book, remember that the title is *It's Not Your Fault*. I selected this title because, if your child is having a toilet training problem, I want you to remember that it's not your fault. It's not your fault because you did not do anything wrong, and it is likely that no one ever told you what you needed to know in order to train your child properly. It's not your fault if no one ever told you what to do if a toilet training problem occurred in your child.

You will learn in this book that your child is not having these problems because he or she is "lazy" or "acting out." Your child does not want to have these potty training issues, but he or she may just not be able to train from a developmental standpoint. This book will help you understand what's going on so you can direct your energy on making the problem go away, rather than focusing on things that don't matter and can be potentially hurtful.

I don't really want to spend much more time on my background, but I do feel it is important to at least briefly describe myself to you.

I want to share my experience with you so that you understand that this book is based on years of scientific and clinical experience and not just my personal opinion or another review of the information that is available on the Internet. This book contains unique information that has not yet been published and is not readily available to the public. I hope that you will be able to use the information in this book to successfully toilet train your child or to fix your child's existing toilet training problem. I have no doubt that, if you read this book, you will have a better understanding of toilet training and toilet training problems in children than many doctors.

Joseph G. Barone, MD
Professor and Chief, Division of Urology,
    Rutgers–Robert Wood Johnson Medical School
Chief of Pediatric Urology and Surgeon-in-Chief,
    The Bristol-Myers Squibb Children's Hospital at
    Robert Wood Johnson University Hospital

To make an appointment, please call 732–235–8853.
The Division of Urology website is at www.rwjurology.com.
You can follow the Division of Urology on Twitter at www.twitter.com/rwjurology.
Please join my network on LinkedIn at www.linkedin.com/in/baronejg.

ABOUT THIS BOOK

This is an evidence-based book on toilet training and toilet training problems. So what exactly does that mean? It means that the information that is contained in this book is backed by scientific studies and is therefore the best information that we have on the topic. Evidence-based information is not easily available on the Internet or in most books; it tends to be found in medical and scientific books and journals. Sometimes it can be difficult to understand, so in this book I would like to provide this information to you using language free of medical jargon.

Most of the information that is readily available to you on potty training is based on someone's personal experience or advice. Maybe someone used one method of toilet training for his child that worked, or maybe a doctor prefers one method of toilet training for her patients. This kind of information is just plain old advice that is not based on any kind of study. Just because it worked for them does not mean it is going to work for you. If we consider evidence-based information, it is more likely that that information will work for most people, including you.

I have organized this book into several logical chapters. The first chapter provides you with the basic information that you need to know about your child's urinary system. I tried not to get too scientific here, and I hope it is fun reading for you. I decided to put this chapter first because it provides you with the basic information you need to know to understand the rest of this book and to toilet train your child successfully.

The second chapter is really exciting because it will help you learn how to toilet train your child using the latest available evidence-based information. This is an extremely important part of the book, and I am really thrilled to be able to share this information with you. I recommend only the best information available, and I make sure that this information is backed by scientific study. This means that the information is evidence-based, high-quality information for your child.

In the third and fourth chapters I discuss common potty training problems that can occur in some children, bedwetting and daytime wetting. These problems occur when toilet training is not totally successful. Let's face it, nothing in life is perfect, so we need to know what to do if a child does not toilet train as well as we had wished. These valuable chapters will provide you with the hope and guidance needed to overcome any toilet training problem.

In the fifth and sixth chapters, I discuss medications and common tests that doctors order for children with persistent potty training problems. Testing and medications are not needed for most children with potty training problems, but I would like you to have this information, just in case. I want to share all of my knowledge with you.

To get different perspectives on the topics discussed in this book, I interviewed three other experts in the toilet training field, and in the seventh chapter I provide you with their takes on the subject. Each expert shares a slightly different viewpoint based on her unique background in public health, pediatrics, and nursing. I am certain you will enjoy reading what these experts have to say about toilet training.

Finally, I conclude with a chapter on alternative treatments for toilet training problems and a chapter covering the most common questions I am asked by parents. I include the chapter on alternative treatments because I want you to know that there are options for potty training problems that most doctors are not familiar with. But I have been careful to include only those alternative treatments that might be beneficial for your child. But most of these alternative treatments have not been studied scientifically, so we can't consider the information in this one chapter to be evidence-based information.

Throughout the book, you will see highlights called "Dry Spots." These "Dry Spots" are meant to draw your attention to the most important potty training information that is available anywhere. Most of this information is missing from the vast majority of potty training books on the market, which I find amazing. When you come across a "Dry Spot," please take a little extra time to read that information and reflect on it. All "Dry Spot" information is backed by science, which means that it is highly accurate and is the kind of information that you can trust for helping your child.

And one more thing: throughout the book I have switched between using female and male pronouns when I talk about children and toilet training and continence problems—it's less clunky than saying "he or she" or "him or her" for each example. But please remember that both boys and girls can have toilet training and incontinence problems.

So let's begin with the first chapter, which discusses the different parts, or ingredients, of your child's urinary system that are needed for potty training. I truly hope you will enjoy this book, and please feel free to contact me with any questions or comments that you might have about this book or potty training.

It's Not Your Fault!

1

TOILET TRAINING INGREDIENTS

Understanding Your Child's Urinary System

I always was a firm believer in understanding the basics of anything we are trying to learn more about. We would not be able to bake a tasty, moist, delicious chocolate cake if we did not understand some basic units of measurements, like what a cup, pinch, or teaspoon is. Imagine how terrible a cake would taste if the recipe called for a a pinch of salt but we used a cup instead. Likewise, how could we help our child with the toilet training process if we don't have a basic understanding of what makes toilet training possible in the first place?

In this chapter we are going to discuss the different parts of the urinary tract and especially learn about the parts that are needed for potty training. We will learn about the kidneys, ureters, bladder, and the stopper muscle that control urination. These are all the ingredients that are needed for successful toilet training, just like flour, sugar, and chocolate are needed in order to bake a tasty cake. After you learn how all of these ingredients come together to make potty training possible, you will be in a better position to understand how to potty train your child and how to deal with any potty training problems that might develop later.

The Journey of a Drop of Water

Water and urine are big ingredients in the toilet training process. Potty training is all about making sure that urine goes into the potty at the right time and place. Basically, water comes into your child's

1

body when she takes a drink or eats food. That exact same water eventually will find its way into the potty. The trick is to get it to go into the potty at the correct time. Your body transforms all water that is drunk into urine, so the more you drink, the more urine you will produce. But here is something that you might find interesting: if you don't drink anything, your body will still make some urine. Because of this fact, you will eventually become dehydrated, or dried out, if you don't drink because your body will still produce small amounts of urine no matter what.

When we potty train our children, we want the urine produced to come out when it's supposed to and not at other times, like when your child is at school or sitting on the new sofa you just purchased. So if your child drinks a lot of water during the day, or before bedtime, then that water is going to have to come out, and it will possibly come out at the wrong time and place.

Dry Spot It makes good sense to avoid fluids two hours before bed to reduce the risk for bedwetting.

After your child drinks fluid, that fluid is sent on to the kidneys for processing, to be turned into urine. It does not matter if your child drinks milk, juice, or water; the body will eventually turn the liquid consumed into urine. So a cup a milk before bed is not any different than giving your child a cup of water before bed. Both milk and water are liquids, and the kidneys will turn those liquids into urine. Since the kidneys are the organs that will transform liquids into urine, we need to understand a little about the kidneys to understand potty training and potty training problems.

The Kidneys

The kidneys are two bean-shaped organs located on each side of your child's back. They are essential ingredients for toilet training. The kidneys are very smart, and they can determine exactly how much water should be kept in the body and how much is excess water that needs to leave the body in the form of urine.

The amount of urine that needs to stay in the body depends on many different things, such as the size of your child, if your child is sweating, or if your child is playing hard at a sporting event. If your child is active and sweating, the kidneys will preserve water so the body does not become dehydrated. If the body loses too much water and becomes dehydrated, bad things can happen, like headaches and even fainting. This is why we want children to drink plenty of water when they are active, especially if it is hot outside. They need to stay hydrated in order to prevent problems from developing.

To keep your child healthy, you should encourage your child to drink water during the day. This is sometimes hard to do because children don't always have access to water at school and they have active schedules, running from one event to the next. And many schools don't allow children to have a water bottle at their desks, and some schools are stingy with bathroom breaks, too. In some cases, things can be so bad that I will write a note to the school nurse requesting that a child be allowed to have a water bottle on his desk to prevent dehydration.

How Much Water Should My Child Drink?

This is a question that parents often ask. The right amount of water to drink depends a lot on the size and age of your child and how much exercise she is doing, but I want to give you a rough guide to follow. If your child is between two and three years of age, one pint of water per day should be fine. If your child is between four and eight years of age, two pints of water a day should be a good baseline. If your child is between nine and sixteen years of age, you probably want to double that amount and encourage your child to drink four pints of water a day. These are general guidelines that can give you an idea about how much water your child should be drinking. A few pints of water per day is not a lot when you think about it, but many children are not big water drinkers, and getting children to drink even this limited amount might not be easy.

Now, if it is very hot outside and your child is playing sports or exercising, you will want to increase that amount to keep your child hydrated. You might even have to double the amount. But how else can you tell if your child is drinking enough water and is not dehydrated? Well, here are a couple of things you can look at. First, you can determine if your child is drinking enough water by looking at his urine. If the urine is clear or light yellow, without an odor, then chances are your child is drinking enough water. If it is dark yellow and smelly, more water is needed! Second, your child should not have a dry mouth. If your child's mouth is dry, then chances are more water is needed. And, third, your child's skin should be supple and soft and not dry.

However, you don't constantly have to monitor how much water your child drinks down to every ounce. You should just have a general idea of the volume of liquid that your child drinks in a typical day. The reason you don't have to worry too much about the exact amount your child is drinking is because the kidneys are like little computers that can figure out how much water needs to stay in the body and how much should leave. Just like you might monitor the water quality in your pool with one of those little dipsticks, the kidneys will constantly monitor the water quality in the blood. The kidneys constantly test the blood, and if the blood has too much water in it, the kidneys will take the water out of the blood by making more urine. If there is not enough water in the blood, the kidneys will preserve water.

So let's look at the kidneys in action. As an example, if it's very hot outside and your child is not drinking enough water, the kidneys will test the blood, and the kidneys' test strip will come back saying, "There is not enough water in the blood." In that case, the kidneys will say, "We need to conserve water, and no more water is leaving the blood!" The kidneys will save every drop of water it can to prevent dehydration, and only a very small amount of urine will be produced. Remember, even if we stop drinking the kidneys will still make a small amount of urine. But this is not healthy. The kidneys run on water, just like a car engine runs on oil. We all know what will happen to a car engine if there is not enough oil in the engine. The engine will continue to run for a while, but it will eventually shut down. Likewise, the kidneys will run for a time without water, but they will eventually shut down if they have to run for a long time without water. This is called kidney failure, and we never want that to happen. That is why it is important to drink a normal amount of water during the day and to increase that amount during periods of increased activity. We want to keep your child's kidneys healthy and strong, and we can do this by providing them with sufficient water to run on.

The Ureters

I am just going to mention the ureters only briefly because they are not really involved in potty training. They are kind of like those "optional ingredients" in recipes that can be left out if desired. But I do want you to at least know what the ureters are. Once a kidney makes urine, the urine flows down a little strawlike tube called the "ureter." The ureters do not have any particular function other than to move the urine from the kidneys into the bladder. Since the ureters are just innocent bystanders in all of this, let's just remember what they are and move on to the main ingredient in our potty training recipe, the bladder. The bladder is really important in the overall potty training process, and if you understand the bladder, you will be able to understand why your child might be having a potty training problem.

The Bladder

The main ingredient of the toilet training process is the bladder. If you want to potty train your child successfully, or if your child is having a potty training problem, you need to understand the bladder. The bladder is like a storage container for the urine. Think of it as like a balloon. As urine enters the bladder, the bladder expands to hold more urine. And, like most balloons, the bladder can only hold a certain amount of urine, depending on how big it is. For example, if your child's bladder is small, she will only be able to hold small amounts of urine. She may not be able to hold urine for two to three hours, like other children. This is an important point to understand.

Table 1.1 The Ingredients of Your Child's Urinary System	
Ingredient	Function
Kidney	Makes urine
Ureters	Carry urine to bladder
Bladder	Stores and empties urine

As the urine flows into the bladder, the bladder will slowly fill until it can't hold any more urine. At that point, your child will either go to the potty, or the bladder will just empty on its own and your child will have an "accident." The bladder, including its size, is therefore a very important ingredient in the overall potty training process. If the bladder is small, then your child may have to go to the bathroom very often. Or, if your child's bladder is big, he may be able to hold urine for much longer periods of time. I have lots of patients who go to the bathroom every hour because their bladders can't really hold much urine and other patients who might go only a few times per day. If you understand the bladder, you can understand why some children can hold a lot of urine while others have to constantly go to the bathroom.

We sometimes say that the bladder in children who go to the bathroom all the time is too small. But we don't consider a small bladder to be a medical problem; instead, we consider it to be a developmental delay. This just means that your child's bladder has not grown along with the rest of him. But rest assured that, as your child grows, the bladder will eventually enlarge to a normal size and will catch up. So having a small bladder is not a terrible thing, and it is not a medical problem.

But I would like you to focus on this point: the size of your child's bladder can determine how easy it is to potty train. If your child's bladder is small and can hold only a small amount of urine, it won't take long before it is filled and your child has to go potty. In this case, your child will need to go to the bathroom more often than other children. A small bladder could make it more difficult to potty train because your child may not be able to hold one or two hours' worth of urine without having an accident.

How to Determine Your Child's Proper Bladder Size

You can determine how big your child's bladder actually *is*, and you can also calculate how big it *should* be. The first thing you will need to do is to have your child urinate into some type of container that will measure how much urine he can hold. Something like a measuring cup will do. When you do this, you have to make sure that your child actually has to go to the bathroom and that the bladder feels full to your child. Take four measurements, in ounces, over the course of a few days and determine the average amount of urine recorded. To determine the average amount of urine recorded, just add up all of the volumes you recorded, and then divide that number by four. It's that simple. This number is a good estimate of your child's actual bladder size.

 Dry Spot Age plus two is the normal bladder capacity for your child in ounces. Compare this to the average volume you obtained. This will help you to determine if your child has a small bladder.

Now that you know what your child's bladder size is, you can determine if it is normal, small, or large. You can determine if your child's bladder size is normal by comparing the average volume that you calculated to the normal bladder size for a child based on age. The formula for determining the normal bladder capacity based on age is simply the age of your child plus two. This gives you the normal bladder capacity in ounces. For example, a five-year-old child should have a seven-ounce bladder capacity (age five + two = seven ounces), and a seven-year-old should have a nine-ounce bladder capacity (age seven + two = nine ounces). Once a child reaches about eight years of age, the bladder capacity is ten ounces (age eight + two = ten ounces), and this represents maximum bladder capacity for most children and young adults. So all children ages eight and above should have a ten-ounce bladder capacity, since the bladder size does not increase much beyond that.

The Urinary Stopper Muscle

There is another ingredient involved with potty training that is important for urine control. In order for the urine to stay inside the bladder, the bladder has to have a way to hold in the urine. Think of the balloon again. If you blow a balloon up but don't tie it closed at the neck, then all of the air will rush out. Well, in order for the urine to stay inside the bladder, something called the "urinary sphincter muscle" has to be working properly to prevent the urine from running out of the bladder, just like air would rush out of a balloon. So in addition to being the proper size, the bladder also has to have a strong urinary sphincter muscle to prevent the urine from leaking out. In this book, I refer to the urinary sphincter muscle as the "stopper muscle."

In some children, this muscle might not work very well; it's kind of leaky, and the urine will sometimes drip out of the bladder when it's not supposed to. I think you can see how this type of leakage might have nothing to do with the bladder size. The bladder could be a normal size, but if the stopper muscle is not working well, the bladder never really has a chance to fill up all the way before it starts to leak. Having a weak stopper muscle could also make potty training more difficult.

If a weak stopper muscle is preventing potting training, then we need to try to make the stopper stronger and work more effectively. We use our own stopper muscles all the time without knowing it. It is the muscle that we use when we have to go to the bathroom but there is no bathroom available—we clamp down on our stopper muscle to keep the urine in the bladder. We don't just urinate on the floor whenever we get the urge to go; we hold onto the urine by squeezing the stopper muscle, and this prevents urination until a bathroom is available.

Understanding how the stopper muscle works may help you understand why its possible for your child to have a perfectly normal sized bladder but still have potty training problems. In this case, the bladder might be normal size, but the stopper muscle is not working very well and can't keep urine in the bladder when it is supposed to. You can get a clue that your child's stopper muscle might be weak if the size of his bladder is normal but he is having trouble potty training.

Review of the Basics

We have learned a lot so far about the different ingredients that are necessary for potty training. Let's take a second to review the recipe briefly. We learned that the first ingredient, water, is turned into urine by the kidneys. The kidneys, our second ingredient, make urine based upon how much water is in the blood and how much water your child drinks. The kidneys send the urine down to the bladder, the third ingredient, through tubes called "ureters," the fourth ingredient. Once the urine reaches the bladder, the urine is stored until it's time to urinate. We learned that, in order for the bladder to hold urine, two things have to happen. One, the bladder has to be a normal size to hold a normal amount of urine. And two, the stopper muscle, the fifth ingredient, has to be strong to hold the urine inside the bladder. That's about it. That is all you really need to know to understand potty training. Now that we understand the basic ingredients of potty training, it is time to start cooking.

2

TOILET TRAINING

What You Need to Know to Toilet Train Your Child Successfully

Now that we understand the parts of your child's urinary system that can affect successful potty training, we can begin to focus in on potty training. Potty training is a process, and it is important that your child be ready to start this process from a physical and mental point of view. In order for potty training to work, your child has to be willing to potty train, and your child has to be mature enough to potty train from a developmental standpoint.

We talked about the different ingredients that are part of your child's urinary system in last chapter. All of these ingredients have to work together in a coordinated fashion if potty training is going to be successful. And it is your child's nervous system that connects all of these different parts together, like spokes on a wheel, which means that these parts, interconnected by the nervous system, are controlled by the brain, and your child's brain has to be mature enough to be able to coordinate and control them.

When a child is very young, the brain is simply not capable of controlling all of these parts because it is not mature enough. As your child matures, the brain slowly begins to be able to control all of the different parts of the urinary system that need to be coordinated for successful potty training. In most children, the brain begins to reach this stage of maturity at around eighteen months of age. However, it is important to note that some children mature more slowly than others, and this developmental delay could slow successful potty training. There is nothing wrong with children who develop, or mature, more slowly than others; they will eventually catch up.

Why Is Development Important for Toilet Training?

A child needs to be able to know when to urinate and when to hold it. Then all of the different parts, or ingredients, of the urinary system need to work together for potty training to be successful. The command center for coordinating this activity is the brain. The brain acts like the conductor of a band, telling the child when, and when not, to go potty and coordinating the different parts to work correctly. When a child is very small, her brain does not really have the ability to control the different parts of the urinary tract, and she will just go potty whenever she wants to.

A baby may urinate twenty or thirty times a day, and this is perfectly normal. If a baby is in the middle of a fine restaurant, the baby will go potty and could care less if the restaurant has been rated four stars. For an older child, however, as the child's brain matures, it will gradually be able to control potty time by controlling the different parts of the system that are responsible for potty training. The brain will eventually tell the child when she should go potty, and it will instruct her bladder and urinary stopper muscle to hold on until she reaches a bathroom.

This developmental process is a natural progression of events that occurs as a child matures. You can probably now see that, if the child does not mature at the normal speed, or if she has subtle developmental delays, then the brain will have a harder time controlling the different parts of the urinary system, and potty training might be delayed. Without the brain controlling things, the child will continue to go potty without regard for time or place. She is not doing it on purpose; her brain is just not in full control yet. It's no different than having a baby's bladder, and we actually call this an "immature bladder."

This is why we sometimes see potty training problems more often in children with other types of developmental delay. Sometimes the developmental delay can be obvious, like a learning deficiency. But sometimes it can be very subtle, like a slight delay in learning to walk or talk. These subtle delays are nothing to be worried about; they simply represent delayed maturation of the nervous system and brain. As the child matures, the brain will eventually gain better control over the potty training process.

It's important to understand this whole developmental issue. Most children with potty training problems and those who are difficult to potty train lack brain control over potty training to some degree. This means that it is very hard for them to control potty time because they are not ready to do so from a developmental viewpoint. They often have accidents because their brains are not mature enough to control things. It's not their fault; they just don't have the ability to control their bladders or the other parts of the urinary system. But don't worry. As they mature, their brains will gain control, and they will be potty trained. Just remember that it's not their fault, and they are not having accidents on purpose.

The Evidence behind Breastfeeding and Development

We did some important scientific studies to determine why some children are potty trained faster than others. In one particular study we looked at breastfeeding and potty training success. We did this study because breastfeeding provides some very important fatty acids in the diet that we just cannot get from formula, even when the formula is fortified. These fatty acids help the development of the nervous system and brain and allow children's nervous systems to mature more quickly, compared to children who are not breastfed. In this study, we compared potty training success in children who were breastfed to those who were fed formula. We found that children who were breastfed had lower rates of potty training problems than children who were fed formula. We believe this is because breast milk allows the child's nervous system to develop better and faster than formula.

The conclusion of our study was that, if you breastfeed your child for at least three months, you will lower the risk of your child developing potty training problems later on in life. So breastfeeding is something that you can do to prevent potty problems in your child, and this recommendation is backed by evidence-based research. This means that we tested this advice using science, and it is not based upon personal opinion alone.

> **Dry Spot**
>
> Breastfeeding during the first three months seems to provide a protective effect against the development of potty training problems later on in life. This is the only known preventative measure against potty problems, and it is evidence based.

Evidence-Based Potty Training Information

There is a lot of not-so-accurate, non-evidence-based information out there about toilet training, so you need to be really careful about what you believe. As I said before, evidence-based advice is based on scientific studies, not personal opinion. When information is based only on personal opinion, that information may not be correct; in fact, the information can sometimes be harmful. One time a parent asked me if it was okay to toilet train their three-month-old because she read an article on infant toilet training. Sure enough, if you look online, you can find "experts" who will give you instructions explaining how to train your infant. But just because you can find information for something on the Internet does not necessarily make that information correct or reliable.

Just remember that anyone can put anything on the Internet. Just because the information is out there and in published format, does not make it true. The best advice is advice that is based on scientific studies, and this is why I am so focused on providing you with only evidence-based advice. I know I have talked about this several times already, but it's a very important point that I want to make sure we agree on.

So how much evidence-based information is available to parents on potty training? Truth be told, not so much. If we go all the way back to the 1930s, we will find fewer than twenty good, scientific articles on toilet training. Can you believe that? Toilet training is one of the most important milestones in a child's development, and there are hardly any good studies for parents to hang their hats on. Compare that to the thousands of articles on other medical issues in children, and we can sense that potty training gets little respect from scientists. It's too mundane, too common, too unimportant, apparently. Well, I don't think so. That is why I decided to begin to study this topic scientifically—so I could obtain some really good information that parents could use to better potty train their child.

I am excited to communicate with you all of the evidence-based information that is available on toilet training and also to share my research on this topic. I will steer you away from things that don't work and from those things that are potentially harmful for your child. My goal is to keep us focused on only the evidence-based information that you can safely use to potty train your child successfully.

> **Dry Spot**
> Potty training is a simple process. It does not need to be difficult or complicated. It may seem complicated, but that's just because there is too much non-evidence-based information out there on the topic.

I would like to describe to you the history of potty training. I think you will find this topic very interesting. And understanding the history of potty training will help us better understand where we are now in terms of potty training advice and knowledge. As the old saying goes, it's important to see where you were in order to understand where you are. Once you see where we were in terms of potty training, and how we got to where we are, you may want to go about toilet training your child differently from what most potty training books recommend.

The History of Potty Training

In the 1930s, the average child was completely toilet trained by eighteen to twenty-four months. That may surprise you because today the average age is closer to thirty-six months. So what happened? Where did we go wrong? Well, to understand why children are being trained much later today than they were over eighty years ago we have to learn a little bit about a great pediatrician named Dr. Benjamin Spock. This is not the Mr. Spock of *Star Trek* fame but a pediatrician who was considered to be the main pediatric expert many, many years ago.

Here is what happened. In the 1930s, when Herbert Hoover was president, the government recommended that children be toilet trained by eighteen months of age. Can you believe that! The U.S. government was actually concerned about when children potty trained. Of course, a government official did not come into the house to check if a child was out of diapers at eighteen months, but the general push was for parents to train children early. Parents were advised to begin toilet training after one year of age and to have it completed by eighteen to twenty-four months. Because parents took charge of the toilet training process and directed it, this method of toilet training was called the "parent-directed method of training." Makes sense to call it that, right? This method says that it is the parents who decide when to start the toilet training process. It's a parent-directed method. The interesting thing about this method was that it was very successful! By using this method, most children were potty trained by eighteen months of age.

This government push for parent-directed potty training led to children being trained early, very early. Maybe they were being trained too early. Remember that, in the 1930s, children were potty trained, on average, by eighteen months of age. That means that, by eighteen months of age, most children no longer needed diapers. What a relief and what a success story! But before you get too excited—keep reading.

If we fast-forward to 2013, the average age of toilet training is thirty-six months, and the number of children who have long-lasting toilet training problems, like wetting their pants during the day, is rising. What in the world happened? Is this an area in child-care where we have gone backward? Did we do something wrong?

Well, yes and no, but I need to explain how it all happened so you can understand where we are now.

Why Are Children Potty Training So Late?

Here's what happened. In the late 1940s, a pediatrician named Dr. Benjamin Spock said he was seeing a large number of children in his practice with constipation. Children were all backed up with poop. You have to understand that Dr. Spock was the most respected pediatrician of his time. You should also know that, at that time, doctors could say things that were not necessarily backed by scientific studies or research. That means that their advice was often not evidence based, and, as a result, many of their suggestions turned out to be partially incorrect.

During the time Dr. Spock saw all of these kids coming to his office with constipation, he wrote a book called *Baby and Child Care* about how parents should raise their children. At the time, that book was the second best selling book of all time. It ranked second only to the Bible! It was such a successful book that it changed the way parents raised their children and how pediatricians guided them.

A big part of the book was about potty training, and the information contained in Dr. Spock's book was what caused parents to start training children later and later, until today the average age of training is up to thirty-six months. Dr. Spock felt that children were being potty trained too early and that constipation was their way of fighting back in protest. He thought that if you trained children to hold their pee at such a young age, then they would hold their poo, too. He felt training before eighteen months was just too early— and he was right.

Training too early was causing constipation, and we can't have that! The message from Dr. Spock was loud and clear: If you are a good parent, you will not potty train your child early. Dr. Spock said that parents should not direct potty training; instead, they should wait until the child shows interest in training. This was a major change in the way parents toilet trained their children. Suddenly, it was the child who was in charge. The child was now directing the toilet training process. As you have probably guessed, this change gave birth to the child-directed method of toilet training.

This method of training began to spread like a virus, and it continues to spread even today. And, because some children have no interest in training, the average age of training has gradually increased from eighteen to thirty-six months. Let's face it, if you are going to wait for your child to give you the green light before you begin training, you could be waiting a very long time.

But think about this for a moment. Dr. Spock's advice was really just not to start training too early. He wanted to avoid constipation. He wanted children to train a bit later than eighteen months, and he said parents should wait until the child gives the green light. I think we ran into problems with this advice because parents did not know what to do if the child never gave them the green light to potty train. So Dr. Spock had good advice—to train later than eighteen months—but parents did not know how long they should wait for training to begin or when the ideal time to begin training was.

Let's now discuss the parent- and child-directed methods of toilet training. We will also learn how to spot signs of toilet training readiness. Like it sounds, these are signs that your child might show that suggest she is ready to begin the toilet training process. All of the information we present will be evidence based and is therefore the best and most reliable information that we have for your child on this topic. You should demand nothing less for your child.

Table 2.1. Average Age of Toilet Training Completion, 1930–2013	
Year	Average Age of Toilet Training Completion
1930	18 months
1950	24 months
1980	27 months
2013	36 months

Dry Spot Advice is based on someone's personal opinion may not be reliable. Facts are based on scientific evidence and are more reliable.

The Parent-Directed versus Child-Directed Method of Toilet Training

As I mentioned, in the 1930s, parents were doing what is called "parent-directed toilet training" without even knowing it. This just means that the parent directed the entire training process and that the child was pretty much a passive participant. The parent decided when to start training, how many times during the day to take the child to the toilet, and how long the child should spend each time on the toilet. Again, this method was very successful and resulted in children being trained at eighteen months of age, on average, back in the 1930s.

Dr. Spock was opposed to the parent-directed method because, in his opinion, toilet training should be child directed. He thought the parent-directed method was pushing children too hard and was causing constipation. He thought it would be a better idea to let the child decide when he was ready to train. This means that the child would direct when toilet training would begin. This approach was a big change from what was being done at the time. In the child-directed method, the child would let the parent know when he had to go, how often he wanted to go, and would even tell the parent when he was ready to begin toilet training. I think you can see why the child-directed method of toilet training would cause children to train later than if the parents took control and started training at a certain defined time. If you use the child-directed method, you have to realize that some children may not have any interest in training and could be three or four years old and still in diapers.

The child-directed method is the most commonly used method of training by most parents today, and I believe that is because it is recommended by the American Academy of Pediatrics. I happen to disagree with this fine organization and believe that the parent-directed approach is better. Maybe someday I can change the academy's mind. The reason I say this is because my research suggests that there is an ideal time to begin training. If you use the parent-directed method, you can begin training during this ideal time. If you use the child-directed method, you could miss out if the child is not ready to train during this ideal time.

The child-directed approach is different from the parent-directed approach in another big way. With the child-directed approach, you don't begin training until the child shows some signs that she wants to begin training. The main problem with this method is that sometimes the child simply does not have any interest in toilet training. Let's face it, some children have no problem staying in a dirty diaper all day. They may not demonstrate signs of training readiness until they are three years of age or older, and at that point they can be quite stubborn, as anyone with a three-year-old or older child knows. I don't think it is in the best interest of the child to wait that long to begin training.

From the time that Dr. Spock wrote his book in the 1940s, there have been arguments as to which toilet training method is better, the parent- or child-oriented approach. To this day, there are proponents on each side, but probably the child-directed method of training is still the most popular. But, just because it is the most popular method, does not make it the best method. In fact, the parent-directed method might have some benefits if we could determine the ideal time to being toilet training. If we knew that there was an ideal time to start training, then the parent-directed method could be used to begin training during that ideal time. Part of my research has been to determine the ideal time for toilet training, and I am now going to share that important information with you.

What Is the Ideal Time to Toilet Train Your Child?

A big part of my research has been to figure out the best time to toilet train a child. This is very important because, if there is an ideal time, it will give you an idea about when to begin training your child. Since the parent-directed method of toilet training is directed by you, the parent, this method of training can be used to start training during this ideal time.

You decide when you want to begin training, when you are going to bring your child to the potty, and how often you are going to bring your child to the potty. You can begin all this during the ideal time. I like this method the best because it is a surefire way to train your child at the best possible time in your child's development. That is because you direct when the training begins.

I can tell you why training your child during this ideal time is important. A few years back, when I did a scientific research study to find out when the best time to begin toilet training is, I thought that knowing the ideal time would give us a better chance for successful toilet training. What I found out was very interesting, and since it is based on science, you can trust it.

I discovered that, if you use the child-directed method and you wait too long to train your child, she will be at higher risk of having problems with toilet training that could persist for many years. I am talking about problems like wetting her pants at school or bedwetting at night. I also discovered that, if you use the parent-directed method and begin to train your child too early, it does no harm—but it may not do any good, either. This means that if you decide to use the parent-directed method and you begin training at twelve months of age, you may wind up taking a longer time to train your child, but in the end you are not doing any harm. So, while we don't want to train too late and miss the ideal time to train, we also don't want to train too early because we could just be wasting our energy and efforts. Let's wait and train during the ideal time.

Dry Spot The ideal time to begin potty training seems to be between twenty-seven and thirty-two months of age.

The ideal time to begin potty training seems to be between twenty-seven and thirty-two months of age, based on my research. Your child will be ready, willing, and able to train at this age during this six-month window of time. If you try to train before twenty-seven months, your child may be too young and may not be able to follow the simple instructions that are needed for potty training. In this case, your overall time spent training will be longer than if you wait until twenty-seven months. If you wait until after thirty-two months to start training, then your child may resist you and begin to fight back against that mean potty because that is the age when they begin to develop independence and a sense of free will. The children who are trained later than thirty-two months are the ones who have the high risk for developing wetting problems that can last years. You want to avoid this by training before thirty-two months of age.

This is why I like the parent-directed method of toilet training. When we use the parent-directed method, it is easy for you to decide to begin training around twenty-seven months, even if she has no interest in potty training. That is what I like about the parent method—you take control. If we use the child-directed method, you might miss out on the ideal time to train if your child does not want to train between twenty-seven and thirty-two months of age.

A large amount of information and advice has been written about each method of toilet training, and thousands of experts have given their opinions about which method is the best. But, what they missed is the "when." It is the "when" that is most important. It is important to begin to train your child between twenty-seven and thirty-two months of age. The "how" is less important. This means that the parent-directed and child-directed methods are both good as long as you begin training during the ideal time period of twenty-seven and thirty-two months of age. If you want to use the parent-directed method, then you just begin training at twenty-seven months. If you feel better about using the child-directed method, then you can begin when you spot signs of toilet training readiness in your child. But if you don't see these signs of toilet training readiness by thirty-two months, use the parent-directed method and just begin. So what are the signs of toilet training readiness that you should look out for in your child?

How to Spot Signs of Toilet Training Readiness

These signs might include things like when your child signals to use the potty, asks to change from a dirty diaper, or wants to imitate big sister or big brother on the potty. Some physical signs of toilet training readiness include some simple things, such as: Is your child able to walk or perhaps even run without falling? Does your child have regular, well-formed bowel movements at regular and predictable time intervals? Do you notice if there are periods of time when your child is actually dry for maybe two hours or when waking up from a nap? These are all physical signs that your child is probably ready for toilet training.

Some behavioral signs of toilet training readiness might include things such as: Can your child sit patiently for a few minutes without losing interest? Is your child able to pull her pants down? Is your child starting to dislike the feeling of a wet or dirty diaper? Children will also sometimes give a physical or verbal cue that they are having, or are about to have, a bowel movement, such as grunting or squatting. Is your child showing signs of being more independent and wanting to do things on his own? Also, is your child showing some interest in using the toilet? If you see the behavioral signs in your child, they are good indications that your child is ready for toilet training.

The studies that I have done demonstrate that, if you wait too long, the toilet training process can be more difficult and there is a

Table 2.2 Signs of Toilet Training Readiness	
Able to sit or walk	Well-formed bowel movements at regular intervals
Can urinate a good amount at a time	Dry period of two hours or more
Can pull pants up and down	Does not like dirty or wet diaper
Shows signs of wanting to be independent	

higher risk for problems like daytime wetting. This is why it might make better sense to begin the toilet training between twenty-seven and thirty-two months of age, even if the child does not demonstrate the classic signs of toilet training readiness. If you think about it for a moment, the child-directed approach to toilet training could potentially delay your toilet training until four years of age simply because the child is unwilling to toilet train. In that kind of situation, I believe it is important for the parent to step in and take charge to begin training using the parent-directed method before it's too late.

So I am not a big fan of the child-directed method because it puts the child in total charge of toilet training. If the child waits too long and decides not to train until after thirty-two months, then that child has just developed an increased risk for wetting problems. We don't let children make other important decisions before age three, so I don't understand why we are willing to let them make this decision. Learning when to use the potty is a big deal, and it ranks right up there with taking the first step in terms of development. That is why I think it is better for parents to take charge of toilet training if the child does not show any signs of toilet training readiness by thirty-two months of age.

In theory, the child-directed method of toilet training sounds nice and child friendly. After all, we are allowing the child to direct the toilet training process and allowing the child to begin when he is ready to train. But in actuality, this method of toilet training has not really worked out very well if we look at the evidence-based advice. This method has resulted in children being trained at much later ages than they were in the past, which leads to more cost associated with diapers, more diapers in our landfills, and more infections in our day care centers. Infections are increased because children who should be toilet trained are instead entering day care centers with dirty diapers.

Before we move on, there is one more thing I want to stress. There is also really no evidence to suggest that the parent-directed method does any harm. It does not seem to cause constipation, as Dr. Spock feared. The only downside of using the parent-directed method too early is that it prolongs the overall time you might spend training. However, by encouraging your child to toilet train at the ideal time, you are actually increasing the chance for successful toilet training in your child.

I would like to mention another form of training called "infant toilet training." This is like the parent-directed method on steroids. You basically use the parent-oriented method but begin very early, sometimes as early as six months of age. I don't suggest this method, but I want you to know that it exists.

The Most Important Thing to Know about Toilet Training

The most important thing to remember about toilet training is to get started and just do it! If your child is younger than twenty-seven months, you can still go ahead and give it a try. You won't hurt anything. It just may take you longer to finish potty training because children younger than twenty-seven months may not be ready to train. So it might take you a little longer, but no harm will be done. If your child is over thirty-two months already, then you need to get started because we don't want any daytime problems later on in life. If you are lucky enough to be reading this book and your child is between twenty-seven and thirty-two months, then you are in perfect shape to start.

If you are expecting, or if you have just had your baby and are reading this book, good for you—because there is something you can do now to make toilet training more successful. We have discovered that there is one thing you can do to reduce the risk for potty training problems in your child. However, you have to do this right after your child is born in order for it to be most effective. Our recent clinical study showed that if you breastfeed your child for the first three months of life, it will reduce the risk for problems like bedwetting when the child is older. The breastfeeding does not have to be exclusive, but it has to be done, and it has to be done early. We think that the fatty acids in breast milk improve the nervous system development that is responsible for toilet training.

I think you know by now that I am a proponent of the parent-directed training method. This method allows the adult to begin the toilet training process rather than relying on the child to determine when potty training should begin. I worry about the child-directed approached toward potty training because the child may not want to toilet train until after thirty-two months of age. If this happens, toilet training might be delayed, and then there will an increased risk of potty training problems.

Does this mean that you should never use the child-directed method? No, it does not. But, if your child does not show any signs of toilet training readiness by thirty-two months of age, just get started anyway. Just do it! Rather than suggesting that you wait a prolonged period of time, I would recommend you start training at the best possible time from a physical and emotional standpoint for the child, and that time is between twenty-seven and thirty-two months of age. What I'm basically saying is that you can use the child-directed method, but just make sure you begin before thirty-two months of age.

Now I want to back up what I am saying with a little evidence-based science because, if I don't back up what I'm are saying with evidence-based information, then how would you know that the advice I'm giving is good advice? In one study my colleagues and I showed that the method of training did not matter. I did another study where I tried to determine if the parent- or child-directed method was better. I looked at the toilet training success in two groups of children. One group was trained using the parent-directed method, and the other was trained using the child-directed method. I discovered that both methods were the same; there was not a big difference in either method. The only thing that was important, once again, was the timing of toilet training. It was important to begin training before thirty-two months if you wanted the most success and least amount of future problems. The method of toilet training used did not matter; what mattered was that you just do it before thirty-two months of age.

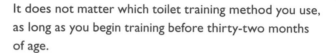

It does not matter which toilet training method you use, as long as you begin training before thirty-two months of age.

Now we know that the most important secret about toilet training success is that you begin training between twenty-seven and thirty-two months. The main difference between the parent-directed and child-directed methods is that, in the parent-directed method, you decide when to begin training, so can begin training during this ideal time. In the child-directed method, the child decides when to begin. I worry about the child-directed method because, if the child does not want to begin training until after thirty-two months of age, then that child will be at higher risk for problems compared to a child who begins training before thirty-two months of age.

So let's assume that we have decided to begin training sometime between twenty-seven and thirty-two months of age because we understand that this is an ideal time to begin training. How do we actually do it? How do we actually toilet train our child?

How to Toilet Train Your Child

The Basic Equipment of Toilet Training

So let's start with a few basics that you will need to have before we get started. First, you will need a comfortable potty chair and a potty seat. The potty chair is your child's own special throne, no one else should have access to it. The potty seat should be portable and should easily go onto and come off of the toilet bowl. Your child may actually grow to prefer this potty to a regular toilet. Another advantage of a good potty seat is that you can take the potty seat with you when you are out and about if you want, or you can just hold your child on a regular toilet seat when you are out.

There are many great potty seats that are available to you and your child. If you look at the Additional Resources section of this book, it will give you a list of places where you can get good-quality potty seats. Look for things like comfort, size, and ease of use when deciding on which potty seat is right for your child. *Parents* magazine did a nice review of the best potty seats, and you can find that article in the Additional Resources section of this book.

If you don't want to use a potty seat or chair, you can use a potty ring. This looks like a small toilet seat, and it fits into a regular toilet seat to make it smaller and more comfortable for the child. You can carry this around with you when you go out, and it's not as big or bulky as a potty chair. The advantage of using a ring is that it gets your child used to using a regular potty, so when he outgrows the ring, the transition to a regular toilet is easy.

Next, you want to get some training pants because we are going to expect some accidents along the way. Training pants are perfect for this use. Parents will often ask me if it is okay to use training pants during the toilet training process. The answer to that question is yes, it is very acceptable to use them. Let's face it, potty training is going to take a few months to do, so let's not be in too much of a rush. Let's take our time, have realistic expectations, and get this done right the first time. Along the way, we can use training pants as needed to make the job easier for everyone—we are not doing any harm when we use them during the potty training process.

We don't want any rashes or abrasions to develop during potty training. So it's a good idea to get some quality wipes to clean your child. You might want to get a plastic sheet for your child's bed because at some point we are going to have to bite the bullet and let your child sleep in his underwear at night.

Positive reinforcement is also going to be important along the way. You might want to stock up on some of your child's favorite stickers or create a reward chart for success. Something as simple as giving your child a star for a job well done could be the motivation that your child needs to get interested in the toilet training process.

So that's about all you need from a supply standpoint. There are probably hundreds of little gimmicks, tricks, and products on the market that you can buy for potty training, but you probably don't

Table 2.3. Basic Toilet Training Supplies	
Potty seat, potty chair, potty ring	Training pants
Wipes	Stickers or stars for positive reinforcement
Books for reading during potty time	Underwear

need them. Save your money and put it in a money market or certificate of deposit for your child's college fund.

Now we will get into the actual steps you should use for toilet training your child. I explain what you need to do and what you can expect along the way. We will discuss the usual order for potty training, so there are no surprises for anyone. Let's get started so we can stop buying those expensive diapers that are taking up all that space in our landfills!

Daytime Potty Training

Children usually gain control along a very predictable pattern. First they gain daytime control, then they gain nighttime control. You should be aware of this pattern and use it to your advantage when training. For example, nighttime urinary control is the last thing your child will master, so we would not want to start out by having your child sleep commando style.

When you begin to potty train your child, start out by having a nice chat with your child and let her know it is time to go potty like a big girl. Let her know that you are going to begin potty training with her and be with her every step along the way. The last thing we want is to make your child feel like she is being punished or that potty training is not fun. We want to focus on praise and rewards for small accomplishments. Your child should be introduced to all the great potty training supplies that you have bought for her. Show her the potty seat and let her play with it, touch it, and sit on it. Let her know that this is her special potty and that you bought it for her because she is a big girl now and that it is time to learn how to go

Figure 2.1   Order of Potty Training in Most Children

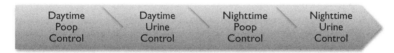

| Daytime Poop Control | Daytime Urine Control | Nighttime Poop Control | Nighttime Urine Control |

potty on this brand-new potty. Introduce her to the Goodnights or training pants that you purchased and let her know that she is going to be wearing these big girl pants while we learn how to go potty. Show her a package of brand-new big girl underpants and let her know that she will soon be wearing these just like a big girl once she learns how to use the potty. In summary, create an atmosphere of fun and excitement about the journey you are about to begin with your child. Take away all fears and eliminate all unknowns as you begin your path down the road to dry days and nights.

Ok, so let's get started. By age twenty-seven months, most children should be able to hold their urine for at least two hours. This is because, at that age, the bladder should be able hold about 120 cubic centimeters, or 4 ounces, of urine. And the average child at age two will usually make about 30 cubic centimeters, or 1 ounce, of urine in two hours. Of course, the more she drinks, the more urine she will make, but your child's bladder should be large enough at that age to handle a two-hour dry period.

Science tells us that the bladder is plenty big enough at twenty-seven months to begin training, and our research also tells us that twenty-seven months is the ideal time to begin toilet training. This is remarkable and excellent news. Now it's just a matter of making the child aware of what a full bladder feels like and letting her know that the feeling of a full bladder is her signal that it is time to go potty. So we can use these evidence-based scientific facts to our advantage as we begin the potty training process.

Dry Spot
The order in which most children potty train should be considered when potty training. First, children develop daytime urine and bowel control, followed by nighttime poop control, and then nighttime urine control.

We begin potty training by taking your child out of the diaper and putting her in training pants instead. Putting her in training pants is important because it sends a powerful message to her that something is different. She is no longer in her diaper and she is wearing something new, but it isn't scary because we have already explained to her what training pants are—and how cool they are!

Next, realize that the clock is your friend. When we start this process, your child is not going to get it right the first time. She won't be able to tell when her bladder is full until she gets the hang of it. This is where you come in. Get a good watch that you can wear, and have it beep or vibrate every two hours. We will begin with the two-hour time interval because a twenty-seven-month-old should be able to hold about two hours' worth of urine before having an accident. If you wait longer than two hours to take your child to the potty, you are asking for trouble. So let's agree to begin by trying to take your child to the potty every two hours.

Use an alarm watch to remind you when it is time for potty. When your watch beeps, this will be your signal to take your child to the potty. Even if your child does not feel like she has to go, or if your child has already had an accident, it is important to take her to the potty every two hours because we are trying to develop good habits and a routine.

When it is time to go to the potty, your child will have to go, no matter what. Take your child to the potty and make sure she is comfortable and place her down on her potty. Use the potty that you bought, the one that you showed her before we started all of this. Once she is on the potty, sit there with her for at least fifteen minutes until she goes. Do not appear rushed, even though you may be. She will sense your urgency, and this will cause her to tense up and make it more difficult to go potty. Sometimes if she is unable to go, try reading a story. After she goes, praise her for a job well done!

If you are unable to have a two-hour dry interval after doing this for seven days, I want you to decrease the time interval by fifteen minutes each day until you start to get dry intervals. For example, if you don't get any two-hour dry intervals after seven days, the next step would be to try taking your child to the bathroom every hour and forty-five minutes. If that does not work, then reduce the interval to every hour and thirty minutes. Eventually, you will find a time interval that your child can manage.

Once you find a time interval that your child can manage to stay dry for during the day, reverse the process until you have achieved a two-hour dry interval. For example, if your child's dry interval is thirty minutes, then stick with that. However, each week, try increasing the potty time by fifteen minutes until you gradually build it up to two hours. What you are doing is stretching out your child's bladder and allowing it to hold more urine each time you increase the potty interval.

Once you are able to make the two-hour mark on a regular basis, continue to gradually increase the potty interval by fifteen minutes each time until your child is dry during the day for three hours at a time. That is our ultimate goal. Once we are consistently dry for three hours at a time, we have mastered daytime urinary control. Keep taking your child to the potty every three hours for two months. Just so you know what to expect, it will probably take you about three months before your child can stay dry during the day on a regular basis for up to three hours, but that is our goal.

Now it's time to back off. Your child can stay dry for three hours, and you have been taking her to the potty every three hours for three months. By this time she should know what a full bladder feels like and has developed excellent potty habits. Your next step is to let your child know that it is time for her to do it on her own. Let her know that you will no longer be telling her when its time to go. Let her know that she is a big girl now and that she has been doing so well that she can now do it by herself. Your role at this point is more like a monitor. Just keep track of what she is doing quietly in the background. Make sure she is going every two to three hours and that she is not going too much or too infrequently. If she is, gently nudge her back into a timed schedule by reminding her when she should go. This monitoring process should continue for about a month or until you are confident that she has mastered daytime control. Once she has gone a month with minimal parental intervention, she is done. She did it with your help and guidance. Your child has mastered daytime urinary control, and you used evidence-based advice to help you achieve your goal. Congratulations on achieving this important developmental milestone in your child's life!

We have been talking about urine control during the daytime, but what about bowel control? In other words, what is the scoop on poop? Well, daytime poop control should be a lot easier to obtain than daytime urinary control. This makes some sense that we can all understand because it is easier to contain a solid compared to a liquid. So how do we achieve daytime poop control in children?

First, be on the lookout for signals that it is time for your child to poop. Here we are looking for signals from your child like grunting, straining, or the famous poop face that most kids make. These are signs of potty training readiness and also are signs that its time for your child to poop. They are signs for you to act on because, if you see your child making one of these signs, poop is about to happen. If you see your child make one of these signs, it's your signal to take her to the potty for poop, even if you are next in line at Wal-Mart on a busy Saturday. You have to do it.

Poop control should be easier than urine control, and you should be able to master it in two months. You just need to figure out when your child usually poops. You probably have a pretty good idea about this already. Most children usually poop after breakfast or dinner. This is because there is a natural reflex in the body that tells the body to poop after eating. This is called the "gastro-colic reflex." As your stomach fills with food, it stimulates your colon to poop. Interesting, right? Make this time, whatever it might be, your child's poop potty time, and be consistent.

Don't try to fight it and make poop time more convenient for you. If your child's natural poop time is 9 A.M., then just deal with it. Trying to change your child's poop time to 5 P.M. because that time might be better for you just won't work. Just go with whatever poop time nature selected for your child. Try taking your child to poop on the potty about the same time every day, and be on the lookout for signs that your child is ready to make poop. Let your child know that this time of the day is her poopy time. Read her a book during poopy time as this will often stimulate the colon to move. You might need to spend up to twenty minutes with your child on the potty before she poops, but you have to be patient. Before long, your child will have complete poop control, all day long. The key is to be consistent and to allow your child enough time to actually poop. Once your child poops, there will be no more poop in the rectum until the same time, next day. This is why you generally will not have poop accidents if your child has a good poop once each day. There is simply no more poop in the rectum to come out.

So we have come a long way at this point in time. We are dry during the day and we are in control of our poop. Now it's time to focus on the night, and we want to be dry all night long, too. This could take a little longer than during the day, so be patient. Most children will get nighttime control by age four, so this phase could happen fast—or it could take a year or even two. So if you have mastered potty training with your child, your child should be pooping once per day and she should be going to the potty every two or three hours to urinate. We might have some accidents every now and then, but if your child is mostly dry during the day and not having many poopy accidents, you are ready for nighttime training.

What about Day Care?

But before we move on to nighttime training, I would like to say something about children who are in day care. If your child is in day care, this doesn't mean that you should delay toilet training. In fact, many day care centers will work with you to toilet train your child because it is also in their best interest to have all of the children in their center trained. This is not only because it is less work for them but because there are fewer infections when everyone is toilet trained at the day care center.

If your child is in day care, ask your day care provider for help during the toilet training process. Most day care centers have a lot of experience in this area and can give you the help you need to toilet train your child while you are away at work or school. For example, it is very common for day care centers to have regular potty breaks, and the teachers are usually very experienced at recognizing signs of toilet training readiness.

So if your child is entering a day care setting and is not toilet trained yet, I would encourage you to speak with your day care provider and develop a plan for your child. You can use the techniques outlined in this book and discuss them with your day care center staff. I am sure they would be very interested in hearing about what your concerns are, and they should be very willing to be your active partner in your child's toilet training process.

Nighttime Potty Training

I am going to let you in on another big secret. You may not like this one, so sit down before you read it. Here it is: There is really nothing you can do before age four to help your child become dry at night. There, I said it and you read it. I hope you are not disappointed in knowing this truth, but it is a fact. You can't really do much before age four to help your child become dry at night.

Nighttime dryness is something that happens automatically. As you "train" your child at night, remember that there is not much you can actually do to stop bedwetting in a toddler. After all, your child is sleeping. This is not like daytime training, where you can take your child to the potty on a regular time interval. For night training, you don't want to wake your child up or take him to the bathroom at night because that won't help stop night wetting and he needs his sleep.

It is normal for a child to sleep through the night and to not have to wake up to use the bathroom by age four. If your child is still bedwetting and has not yet reached age four, there is not much to do about that. The only things I would recommend for nighttime training are commonsense things. First, we will want to put that plastic sheet on the bed that we bought along with our other potty training supplies. Next, we will want to put him to bed in some sort of training pants. It makes sense to avoid diapers, which will suggest to your child that we are expecting dry nights. We should avoid excess fluids two hours before bed, and we will make sure we have one final potty time before going to sleep. This will at least make sure that your child goes to bed with an empty bladder. Limiting fluids before bed will reduce the amount of urine that he makes during the night and is also a good idea.

Then, before he goes to bed, I would encourage you to tell him a bedtime story about how big boys and girls have dry beds and that you are using training pants because he is going to be dry at night soon, too! This is the power of suggestion, and it can be a powerful tool in your nighttime training process. You want your child to start imagining what its like to be dry at night. You can help him visualize this through story telling and reinforce that thought by putting him to bed with training pants on.

There is not much more you can do to help your child become dry at night. At this point, you just need to be patient. I know this may sound like a letdown, but it's evidence-based advice. Don't waste your time, money, or energy trying to follow some unproven nighttime program for a child who has not yet reached the right age. Your main job in achieving nighttime control should be to keep up the nighttime ritual and to not give up hope. If you feel you are not making progress and your child is over four years of age, we need to take an inventory of what we have been doing.

What to Do When Things Go Wrong

In most cases, potty training will be complete by age four. However, for some children it could take longer, and complete potty training will not happen until the child is much older. I have seen some children who are ten years old and are still having problems with daytime urinary control and other children who are getting ready for college and are still wetting the bed. If your child falls into this large group of children, realize that you are not alone and that we can help. Sometimes a formal bedwetting or day wetting treatment program will be needed. For those children, we have sections in this book dedicated to daytime wetting and bedwetting. But before we go there, let's just do a brief review to make sure we did everything according to plan and did not miss any opportunities for success.

When things do not go according to plan, you have to take an inventory to see what potential problems might be preventing successful completion of toilet training. The first thing to do would be to take a break for two weeks and step back and just try to observe your child. Try to see if he is demonstrating any signs of toilet training readiness, try to determine how long he can stay dry, and try to determine when he poops.

We need to figure out if your child has any interest in toilet training. Do you think your child is at all uncomfortable in the diaper? Does your child fight you during the toilet training process, or is your child willing but unable to train? A child who is willing but unable may not be ready from a developmental standpoint to train. If you have been trying and your child seems willing and you are hitting a brick wall, take a break. Taking a break will take some pressure off of your child and will allow your child's body to mature. After a two-to-four-week break you can try again.

If your child is not interested in training, or if your child has been fighting you every step of the way, then it's a different situation. Here it is a battle of wills. In this situation, did you start training late, after thirty-two months? If it is a battle of the wills, it is essential to get your child on your side. You should review all of the toilet training supplies with your child and have a friendly but firm discussion about the importance of toilet training. You want to make total training something positive that is goal oriented and something that he will look forward to, instead of fighting against. You both need to be on the same page if you are going to succeed.

You also need to take an inventory of yourself. Make sure that you are committed to toilet training from a parental standpoint. Are you paying attention to the steps outlined in this chapter for taking your child to the potty on a timed schedule, or are you missing some of those potty times? Are you always willing to make a mad dash to the bathroom regardless of your situation? Even if you are next in line at the grocery store checkout and have loaded all your groceries onto the conveyor belt and there five people behind you? Have you consistently dropped everything to take your child to the potty? Are you doing everything you can as a parent if you are having a difficult time toilet training your child?

Are you consistent with your potty training plan, or are you using training pants and diapers when it is convenient for you? If you are going out to dinner and don't want to be interrupted by having to take your child to the potty, that sends a bad signal to him, one that says potty training is not that important. Do you sometimes just throw the diaper on for convenience's sake? Sometimes we all probably do these things, and most of the time they don't cause any problems or issues. But, if you are having trouble toilet training your child, these small factors can add up and may play a big role in preventing your success. So if you are having difficulty with potty training, take an inventory of what you are doing, and make the changes that you need to make in order to help your child during this process. In the end, you will be successful, and your child will be happier and drier as a result.

But sometimes, despite our best efforts and intentions, children will have ongoing potty training problems. This usually occurs through no fault of our own; remember, the title of this book is *It's Not Your Fault*. That is why I chose that title for the book. Because in most cases where children do not train successfully it is not because the parent or child did something wrong. Rather, it's because of other developmental issues that you have little control over. We will dive deep into these other potty training problems in the upcoming sections of this book. But before we even begin to talk about how to deal with persistent potty training problems like bedwetting and day wetting, we need to now understand a little about how the urinary system works. We need to build your foundation of knowledge so you can not only understand why your child is having a potty training problem but also take steps to help your child, using evidence-based information.

3

BEDWETTING

How to Stop Bedwetting and Become a Bedwetting Slayer!

"Doctor, have you ever seen a fifteen-year-old boy who still wets the bed?" That is a typical question I hear every day from frustrated parents. My usual answer is, "Yes, today I have seen a fifteen-year-old boy, two twelve-year-old girls, and several children under the age of ten, all with the same problem as your son!" Parents often do not realize that bedwetting is one of the most common of all pediatric conditions that exist in children between the ages of five and fifteen years. So take comfort, for you are not alone. No matter how old your child is, there are many, many other children struggling with the same problem.

I just wish people would come in sooner to see me for help because we can stop bedwetting. Unfortunately, many parents don't come in to see me until it is time to send Johnny off to college. The panic sets in when parents begin to wonder about how bedwetting will go over in a crowded dorm room. You don't have to be in that situation if you learn about bedwetting and treat it early. This chapter will help you make the right decision for you and your child and will teach you how to become a certified bedwetting slayer. We don't want anyone going off to college worrying about bedwetting; college is stressful enough, thank you. Bedwetting can be treated and cured, and I am going to show you exactly how to do it.

How Common Is Bedwetting?

So how common is bedwetting compared to other common pediatric conditions? Well, it's bloody-nose-and-earache kind of common! Would you believe that, each year, approximately seven million children ages five and over wet the bed? That's more than the entire population of Switzerland. Talk about yellow snow! With those kinds of huge numbers, it's no wonder that there is such a big demand for childhood diapers, plastic sheets, and other bedwetting products. Companies are waiting in line to make money off of your problem; however, most of the products do not work to stop bedwetting. That is why you need to learn what is in this book so you can slay bedwetting.

Even though bedwetting is common, parents don't usually know much about it. Nobody wants to talk about it. It's like a hidden family secret, in many cases. We keep it quiet, and we typically do not discuss it at lunch. The information that most parents have about bedwetting is therefore usually wrong and potentially harmful. That is why it is important to read this chapter carefully because you won't find this information anyplace else. I have researched dozens of bedwetting books that are on the market, and none has the information that is contained in this book. I can assure you of that fact.

Can Bedwetting Be Treated?

One of the most important things that I want parents to know about bedwetting is that it can be treated without any medicine in up to 90 percent of cases. It amazes me how often parents will bring their child in to see me for bedwetting for the first time as a teenager. At this age, many of the "children" are fully grown and have had to deal with a lifetime of wet sheets and dirty laundry. Imagine how many sleepovers and campouts they have missed and how bedwetting has affected their relationships with friends. The look of sadness and frustration is always clearly visible on a teenager's frowning face when I discuss bedwetting with him for the first time. Amazingly, when I ask parents, "What have you done so far to treat your child's bedwetting?" they typically answer "Nothing." At this stage in the conversation, the teenager continues to look down at his shoes, feeling humiliated. It is sad that this family has had to endure years of wet sheets when they did not have to. When I tell a teenager and his parents that I can cure his bedwetting, the child looks up for the first time during the visit with hope and happiness in his eyes.

Why Do Some Parents Wait So Long to Treat Bedwetting?

When I ask parents why they waited so long to see me, they always say the same thing: "I was told my child would outgrow it." Sometimes I want to shout when I hear that kind of advice while looking at a fifteen-year-old whose life has been affected by bedwetting. What a terrible situation, because I know that child could have been treated at age seven and we could have prevented ten years of bedwetting and allowed him to enjoy 240 sleepovers missed during his childhood.

Dry Spot

While it is true that most children will outgrow bedwetting, it typically takes a very long time without treatment. On average, if you wait four years, your child will have a 50 percent chance of continuing to wet the bed at night if you do nothing.

How Long Does It Take to Outgrow Bedwetting?

Why would anyone, especially a doctor, tell you that your child would outgrow bedwetting? Well, because that statement is true and accurate. I just don't think it's good advice. What is missing in that advice is how long will it take for the bedwetting to stop. Let's do some simple math to illustrate the point. At age five, about 15 percent of all children wet the bed. This means that if we take one hundred random five-year-olds from kindergarten classes in any school district, fifteen of those hundred children will have a bedwetting problem. So, if your child is in kindergarten or first grade, he is not the only one wetting the bed in the class; there are others. You just don't know who the other kids are because nobody likes to talk about bedwetting! What a shame, because the only way we learn is to share our ideas and experiences.

But let's say we take the advice of our friends and family and do nothing about bedwetting but wait five long, wet years for it to go away. If we now go to any sixth-grade class and look at a hundred children, about ten of them will still be wetting at night. In those five long years, only five children stopped wetting! Those odds are not very good.

But let's say we are really, really patient and we decide we still want to continue to wait and do nothing about bedwetting. We continue to believe that our child will outgrow bedwetting, as we were told. Now our child is in high school, and if we go into any high school and look at a hundred children aged fifteen years, we will be amazed to see that one unfortunate child is still wetting. If we multiply that percentage times the estimated number of fifteen-year-olds in the United States, we can estimate that thirty thousand fifteen-year-olds are still wetting the bed. This is not a small number.

Those are the cold, hard facts about outgrowing bedwetting. But, I promise, no more math! I just wanted to show you how common bedwetting really is and how long it can sometimes take to go away on its own.

Figure 3.1   How Common Is Bedwetting at Different Ages?

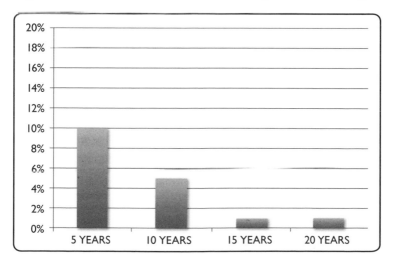

Bedwetting Fact and Fiction

Now that we understand how common bedwetting is, we need to talk about what causes it—all the millions of wet sheets, missed sleepovers, and ruined mattresses. The good news is that science has a pretty good idea why children wet the bed. As a pediatric urologist and researcher, I have helped discover this scientific information, and I have used it to develop a foolproof treatment plan for children who wet the bed. My method is based on scientific research and medical experience, not guesswork or intuition.

Before I talk about the method I use, I would like to bring up some of the more common facts and fictions about bedwetting. I think this is important because there is so much bad information out there. I don't want you following bad advice, and I have seen bad advice on some pretty reputable websites. You need to know what is right and what is wrong so you can make the best decision for your child and family.

Dry Spot Bedwetting is very common, and while it can stop by itself, it can take a very long time to go away. There is no guarantee that it will stop, even if you wait until your child is fifteen years old.

FACT OR FICTION #1
Boys wet the bed more than girls.
This is a fact. Boys are about twice as likely to wet the bed than girls. We are not really sure why this is, but it probably has to do with the fact that girls tend to mature faster than boys.

FACT OR FICTION #2
There are no risk factors for bedwetting.
This is fiction. By far, the most important risk factor for bedwetting is a family history of bedwetting. If one parent wet the bed, the child has a 20 percent chance of wetting the bed. If both parents wet the bed, the child has a 40 percent chance of wetting the bed. This is probably related to a genetic delay in development that is passed down through families. We will talk about that more in a little bit.

The other big risk factor for bedwetting is snoring. One of my research studies got a lot of national press attention because it showed that children who snored were at high risk for bedwetting. We will discuss it more later, but for now, just remember that, if your child snores, his risk for bedwetting is increased. In the same study, I also found that being overweight is not associated with bedwetting—unless your child snores. Obvious things, like drinking before bedtime and not going to the bathroom before bedtime, are not really risk factors for bedwetting, but they are often considerations in a bedwetting treatment program, and addressing them just makes good sense.

FACT OR FICTION #3
My child wets the bed because he is lazy and does not care.
This is a myth. Children don't wet the bed because they are lazy or don't care. Believe me, your child does not enjoy sleeping in wet sheets or missing summer camp to stay home with dear old Mom and Dad. Bedwetting happens during sleep because the subconscious brain can't tell the bladder to "not go" until the morning.

The subconscious brain is the part of the brain that works without our needing to be aware. It is the brain's autopilot and directs many activities without our thinking about it. One of those activities is bladder control. The bladder is not very smart! If the brain does not tell it what to do, the bladder will let go—and it doesn't really care where you are or what you are doing; it will let go anytime and anywhere.

The bladder always wants to go, and the only thing preventing you from peeing on yourself right now is that your subconscious brain is telling your bladder to "not go" because you are reading a really awesome book. You are not thinking about "not going"; your subconscious brain is doing all the work without your being aware. You are on autopilot.

If the brain can't control the bladder, the bladder will act out like a misbehaving two-year-old. If the bladder is not under good control by the brain, the bladder will empty at night, and bedwetting will happen again and again. Now why doesn't the brain have the ability to control the bladder? This will take a little science to explain, but I am confident that I can explain it clearly.

The brain, which is part of the nervous system, is connected to the bladder by other parts of the nervous system that act like wires carrying messages to the bladder. The brain is on the top, in the head, and the bladder is down below, and the wires connect them. In children who wet the bed, these wires are not fully developed, and when the brain sends messages to the bladder, they may not get through. Think of it like a train trying to get to a railroad station on an unfinished track. The train can't go through until the track is finished. Likewise, the "don't go" signal sent by the brain to the bladder can't get through until the track of your child's nervous system is fully developed.

But relax, nothing is broken; your child's nervous system is just not fully developed or matured. With development, age, and maturity, your child's nervous system will develop, and bedwetting will stop—eventually. This is why it is correct to say that most children will outgrow bedwetting. As the child's neurological track develops, bedwetting will stop. But it may take some time for that track to be built.

Since bedwetting represents a developmental delay, your child may have had other minor delays growing up, such as delayed speech or problems with fine motor skills. These delays also represent simple, normal delays in development, just like bedwetting. As your child develops and matures, she will typically outgrow many of these minor delays. And that's it for the science! I hope it was clear because I really would like you to understand why your child is wetting the bed.

So now you know that when anybody tells you that your child will outgrow bedwetting, what she is really saying is that, as your child's nervous system matures and develops, the railroad track between the brain and the bladder will develop and bedwetting will stop. But now you also know that the process of building that track can be a very slow process that can take many years and there is no guarantee of completion. Fortunately, there are ways that we can speed up track construction, and we will talk about that very soon.

FACT OR FICTION #4

My bedwetting child is a deep sleeper.

This is a fact. Most children who wet the bed are very deep sleepers. An alarm clock can go off, the dog can be barking, and everyone in the house will be awake, except for your child, who will be sleeping soundly in his wet bed. There is no doubt that children who wet the bed are deep sleepers, but I don't want you to confuse deep sleep with abnormal sleep or a sleep problem.

When I do sleep studies on children with bedwetting problems, 90 percent of the time the study is normal. That is because deep sleep is not abnormal; it is just another sign of developmental immaturity. Babies also sleep very deeply. As your child grows, develops, and matures, his sleep will lighten up, and sleep will no longer be so deep. Sleeping lighter will help the brain sense when the bladder is beginning to fill, which will allow the brain to send that "stop" signal

Figure 3.2   The Brain Tells the Bladder to Go When a Bathroom Is Available

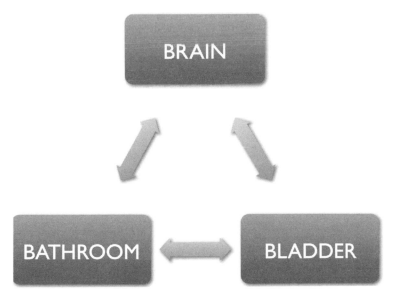

down the nervous system track to stop bedwetting. If your child is a very deep sleeper, the signal will never be sent down the track to the bladder because the brain is not able to sense the bladder filling.

There is one important thing I need to mention at this point. If your child wets the bed, is a deep sleeper, and snores, it *could* be a sign of abnormal sleep. That was part of a research finding I made several years ago. Children who snore and wet the bed may have something called "obstructed sleep apnea." "Sleep apnea" may sound like a big word, but it actually just means that the child temporarily stops breathing at night while sleeping. In addition to snoring, other signs of sleep apnea include gasping for breath at night, restless sleep, and being tired in the morning after sleep. Sleep apnea is important to detect because it can not only affect your child's health but also your child's ability to pay attention and learn at school. Sleep apnea can only be diagnosed by a sleep study that usually involves sleeping in a hotel-type room overnight, so kids love sleep studies. If you think your child has sleep apnea, tell your pediatrician.

A sleep study is not invasive and does not hurt. During sleep, your child will be monitored to see if there are periods where breathing stops temporarily. If breathing stops and the oxygen level in the blood goes down, then your child has sleep apnea. Sleep apnea is fairly common, and is also associated with children who may be overweight. The cause is usually enlarged tonsils or adenoids that block the child's airway when he is lying flat. The obstructed breathing causes the release of a hormone that causes the body to make large amounts of urine at night, and this increases the risk for bedwetting.

> **Dry Spot** Removing the tonsils in a child with sleep apnea will cure the bedwetting in 50 percent of the cases.

Now that we understand the bedwetting basics, we can begin to talk about a medicine-free way to treat the problem. This method is safe and effective in up to 90 percent of children in curing bedwetting. It is not a quick fix, though; it is a cure for your child's lifelong problem. The cure can happen is as little as one month, but two to three months is average. That sure beats the other choice of letting your child "outgrow" bedwetting, which as we now know could take years. Your goal is to cure bedwetting now and cure it fast and become a bedwetting slayer.

So here it is. Here is the big secret to stop bedwetting. Here is what I have learned after practicing twenty years as a pediatric urologist. The best way to cure bedwetting is to correctly use a bedwetting alarm by using my method.

> **Dry Spot**   The best way to cure bedwetting is to correctly use a bedwetting alarm by using my method.

Bedwetting Alarms

You may have heard about bedwetting alarms, but you have not heard about the right way to use them. It's like getting a fancy sports car without knowing what features it has or how to use it. Without understanding how to use the car, the car will only do so much. Sure, you can drive it back and forth to work, but the car is capable of doing so much more. If you are given driving instructions by an expert driver, you will begin to see that your sports car is capable of doing amazing things that you did not realize. I will be your instructor as we drive toward dry nights.

When my method is used properly, it will cure up to 90 percent of children with bedwetting within two to three months. You heard that right! If you use my method correctly, your child is likely to be dry in two to three months. No more wet sheets, no more training pants, no more missed sleepovers. I can quote that success rate because it is based on twenty years of actual results. All you have to do is follow the advice that I share with you in this book.

One of the most important things that you will learn in this chapter is my way to use the bedwetting alarm. I am going to teach you how to slay bedwetting, and you won't be alone in this journey. Anyone can buy a bedwetting alarm on the Internet, but unless you really know how to use it, the alarm probably won't work. It certainly won't be as effective as it could be if you have proper instruction for using it. That is why it is so important for me to explain exactly how the alarm should be used, using my methods. I will provide you with some of the most important tips that I have learned over the last twenty years as a pediatric urologist, tips that will make the alarm more effective and a foolproof cure for bedwetting.

So let's start with the basics. First, what is a bedwetting alarm? It's a very simple device, not as complex as a sports car! A bedwetting alarm has two parts, a sensor and an alarm. The sensor goes inside your child's underwear and attaches with a clip. This part senses wetness. The other part is the alarm, which actually makes a noise. The alarm part is attached to your child's pajamas near the shoulder by a clip. Both parts are very small and won't cause any discomfort for your child at all.

Both parts of the bedwetting alarm, the sensor and the alarm, are connected by a small wire. Wireless alarms exist, but they are not necessary. I generally don't use wireless alarms because they cost twice as much as wired alarms, and they are not any more effective.

Dry Spot

Don't be disappointed if you have already tried a bedwetting alarm and it did not work. Many patients in my practice had already tried an alarm without success. This was not because the alarm was ineffective; it was because the parents were never taught my method.

How Does the Bedwetting Alarm Work?

Here is how the alarm works. When your child begins to wet, the moisture sensor part of the alarm that is in your child's underwear will sense the wetness. There is no shock or pain, it simply senses wetness. The sensor sends a safe signal to the alarm component that is clipped to your child's pajamas. This signal causes the alarm to ring loudly—like an alarm clock. That's it! Pretty simple, right? There is really nothing more to it; it is a very simple device. One part senses wetness, the other part rings like an alarm clock. That is all you need to know about the alarm.

The alarm stops bedwetting by building the nervous system track between the brain and the bladder that we talked about in Fact or Fiction #3. Because the alarm causes the connection from the brain to the bladder to actually develop, it is a cure for bedwetting. Once that connection is built, your child will stop wetting the bed because the signal from the brain will be able to get through to the bladder. This is why using the alarm is a cure for bedwetting, not just a quick fix.

Types of Bedwetting Alarms

There are different types of alarms to choose from, so it is important that you buy an alarm that is going to be effective. I don't want you to waste your money and, more important, I want you to succeed. The most important thing to remember is to get an alarm that makes a noise, a loud noise. There are vibrating alarms, but vibration

Figure 3.3 How Bedwetting Alarms Work

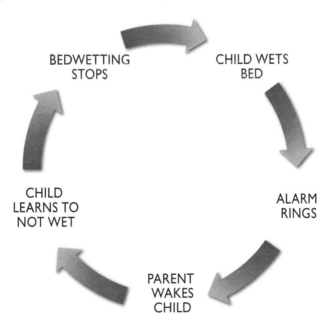

is not good for what we are doing, so stay away from alarms that only vibrate. Some alarms vibrate and make a noise, and those are good for our purposes also. Just make sure you get a good-quality alarm since cheaper units can break and malfunction. Most online stores that sell these alarms will have customer reviews attached to each product, so select one that has great reviews.

The other thing to watch for when you buy an alarm is that the part of the alarm that senses wetness goes *inside* the underwear. This is because we want the alarm to go off the instant your child starts to wet. Alarms with sensors that go on the outside of the underwear or on the bed sheet will take longer to sense the wetness, and they will not be as effective.

Bedwetting alarms can range in price from $60 for a basic model to $200 for a wireless type. You really don't need to spend a lot of money on the alarm; just make sure you buy one that has the features that I mentioned. In my practice, I tend to favor low-cost, readily available alarms that make noise and have moisture sensors that go inside underwear. They are readily available at retail stores and online.

When you get the alarm, read all of the instructions that come with the alarm, but follow the advice in this chapter. If anything in the instructions is different from what I am telling you, go with my advice. It is based on twenty years' experience and a 90 percent success rate!

Dry Spot When purchasing a bedwetting alarm, make sure it makes a noise and that the moisture sensor goes *inside* the underwear.

Bedwetting Alarm Companies

One final word about alarms and alarm companies. There are companies that will provide emotional support for you while you use the alarm. Basically, they will call you periodically to find out how you are doing and will give you a pep talk. There is nothing wrong with this approach, but you don't need it. In fact, after reading this chapter, you will know more than the support counselors used in most of these programs. You will also save yourself over $1,000, which is the typical cost for one of these bedwetting support programs.

Before You Begin to Use the Alarm

Before we get into the nuts and bolts of how to use the alarm using my method, let's talk about some things that will make you less nervous about using the alarm. First, most children will wet the bed an hour or two after they go to bed. This means you won't be waking up at 2 A.M. every night. So be alert during the first few hours after your child goes to sleep and listen for the alarm. Second, you should know that most children wet the bed only one time per night. So relax, you will not be getting up and down all night. You will probably just have to wake up your child once, so do it right and make it count.

 Dry Spot Most children wet the bed only once per night and wet about one or two hours after falling asleep.

Finally, a bit of housekeeping. You can still use training pants to save your sheets while you are using the alarm. There is no reason to make this any harder than it needs to be. Here is what you do. First clip the alarm inside of your child's underwear. Then put the training pants over the underwear. Simple as that! The alarm will still work fine, and your sheets will be saved.

Let's now talk about some common sense things we can do while using the alarm. First, it makes good sense to avoid getting your child overtired during the day, since we don't want him sleeping any more deeply than he already does. Make sure he is getting at least ten hours of sleep each night. You do not need to be concerned that the alarm will make your child tired for the next day. Remember, most children only wet once per night, and they wet soon after they go to bed. When you are using the alarm, your child should still wake up feeling good, and it will not affect his mood, activity level, or school performance. One last point: it is also a good idea to limit fluids two hours before bed and to make sure your child goes to the bathroom before bed. Limiting fluid before bed is just common sense. It is not mandatory, but these things will probably make the alarm work faster and better, so why not do them?

We are getting ready to talk about my method, and I am going to share all my secrets with you. But before we get into that, I would like to make sure that you pick a good time to start using the alarm. It's important that you use it for two or three months straight, with no missed nights, if possible. Try not to start using the alarm if you are going to be going away on vacation or moving in the next few months. Start using it at a time when everything at home is stable (or as stable as it can be!) and when there are no trips or major events planned for the next few months.

Let your child know that he has only two duties when using the alarm. One, he has to agree to wear it every night without any temper tantrums, fits of rage, or crying. Make him sign an agreement so it's official. Two, he has to agree to keep a record of dry nights using a chart. Every time he gets a dry night, he gives himself a star on the chart. Most alarms that you buy will come with a chart and stickers for your child to fill out. Aside from that, your child does not really have to do anything for the alarm to work. The rest of the responsibility is with dear old Mom and Dad. Along the way, feel free to indulge in a reward or two, for you and your child, for a job well done. Small bits of progress deserve a reward!

My Secret Method for Stopping Bedwetting

Now I am ready to share my method with you. Without this method, the alarm has a lower success rate. With my method, you will have a 90 percent success rate of slaying bedwetting in two to three months. I also want you to know that you already know more than most people do about bedwetting, so feel proud about that. You are learning to help your child overcome a big problem!

So here we go. Please pay careful attention to the next few paragraphs. I am about to give you my method for making the alarm

90 percent successful. I will tell you things that most people, even doctors, do not know. I am going to make you a bedwetting slayer. Here is the first bedwetting slayer fact that you need to know when using the alarm: When the alarm rings, it won't wake up your child.

Dry Spot   When the alarm rings, it won't wake up your child.

The number one reason parents tell me that the alarm didn't work is that it didn't wake up the child. Well, guess what? It's not *supposed* to. If the alarm goes off, and your child doesn't wake up, it doesn't mean that the alarm isn't working. All it means is that proper alarm instructions were never given. The alarm may be a simple device, but it is not simple to use.

Is Your Child a Zombie?

Remember I said that children who wet the bed are deep sleepers? They are like zombies! That is one key to slaying bedwetting. I am sure you have tried many times to wake up your little zombie at night, dragging him to the bathroom. A fire truck could pass through his bedroom, sirens roaring, and you *know* that your zombie wouldn't flinch. Why then would we expect a small alarm to wake up a zombie? Well, I don't!

Dry Spot   Most bedwetting zombies are deep sleepers who need help waking up when the alarm goes off.

Ok, so your child isn't a zombie, he's just a deep sleeper. A very, very deep sleeper. We know that. So here comes a bedwetting alarm tip that nobody else will tell you. This tip is essential for you to know and understand if the alarm is going to work. Please stop and think about it for ten seconds after you read it, because it is going to change the way you think about bedwetting alarms: The bedwetting alarm is designed to wake *you* up, not your child.

That's right! When the alarm goes off, it is your signal to go into your child's room and wake him up. How's that for a table turner?

The bedwetting alarm is designed to wake *you* up, not your child.

Trust me, your child won't hear the alarm. He is out cold and won't hear a little alarm going off, even if it is clipped to his pajamas. The alarm is designed to alert *you*, and it is up to you to wake your child up. And when I say, "Wake him up," I mean WAKE HIM UP! No fooling around here, he has to be fully awake for this to work, so don't be shy!

Wake Up Your Zombie

Don't worry about taking your child to the bathroom. Don't worry about changing the sheets. Just worry about just waking your child up. We know that may not be easy, but you have to do it if you want to cure bedwetting and become a bedwetting slayer. If you have to, keep a cold bowl of water next to the bed and wipe your child's face with a washcloth to fully and completely wake him up. I don't know what else I can say to make you understand how important it is to fully and completely wake up your child is during this process. So, now its time for my next tip; stop and think about this for twenty seconds before moving on: Waking your child up is the key to success. If you don't fully and completely wake your child up, the alarm will not work.

 Waking your child up is the key to success. If you don't fully and completely wake your child up, the alarm will not work.

So how can you make sure your child is awake enough for the alarm to work? Here are a few suggestions. First, wake up your child in the bed. There is no reason to get him out of the bed, and it may even be dangerous to stand up a zombie, so leave him where he lies. And don't worry about taking him to the bathroom. Many parents think it is important to get him to the bathroom. It's not; he's already wet! He's already wet the bed! But we don't care about that.

Taking him to the bathroom does nothing to stop the bedwetting, and remember, we are only interested in doing things to stop bedwetting. Just sit him up in the bed and wake him up, right there. Let me repeat that: WAKE HIM UP IN THE BED! So now it is time for another tip. Please stop and think about this one for fifteen seconds before moving on: It does not matter if your child has already wet the bed by the time you wake him up. It just matters that you wake him up.

> **Dry Spot** — It does not matter if your child has already wet the bed by the time you wake him up. It just matters that you wake him up.

That's right. I don't care if the bed is already wet by the time you get into your child's room. That does not matter one bit. What matters is that you wake him up. Don't worry about anything else. Even though he may look like a little wet angel lying there, you have to wake him up. The stakes are high here; we are talking about slaying bedwetting. Second, after you think he is awake, ask him three simple questions: What is your name? What is my name? and Where are you? If he says that his name is SpongeBob, that you are the president, and that he is at a Disneyland, then he's not awake. Try again, and ask him the three questions all over again. Keep doing it until he gives you the correct answers. He eventually will get all three correct. Once he answers all three questions correctly, you should congratulate yourself, for you have woken up the zombie and you are on your way to becoming a bedwetting slayer.

Give Your Zombie a Code Word

Now that your child is awake and alert, and no longer a zombie, let him know that he just wet the bed and that he needs to get changed. No rush, take your time, the bed is already wet. Now you can finally get him out of the bed, take him to the bathroom, and change the sheets on the bed if you need to. Once everything is all cleaned, remember to put the alarm back on him before you lay him down to go back to sleep. One final important point: Before he goes back to sleep you need to give him a code word. Tell him "The code word for tonight is apple" (or something like that). We want to see if he is awake enough to remember the code word in the morning. So the next morning you should ask him two things: Does he remember your waking him up last night? and What was the code word was from last night? If he can answer both questions, then you are on your way to dry nights. If he looks at you like you have three heads and doesn't remember your waking him up, then that whole performance last night was a big waste of time, and we will just have to try harder the next night. Remember to use a different code word every night. I had one parent who used the same code word every night, and the child never guessed it wrong!

As you repeat this process every night, you will see that your child will soon start to wake up by himself when the alarm goes off, and you will soon start seeing some dry nights, typically during the first two weeks. Your success as a bedwetting slayer totally depends on how well you wake him up. Did I mention that waking him up is important? How excited are we if we're talking about dry nights in as little as two weeks after putting up with years of wet beds?

Table 3.1 Secrets to Stopping Bedwetting	
Secret	Why It Works
Get a quality alarm	These things can break
Be consistent	Learning requires consistency
Wake your child up when the alarm rings	No waking means no learning
Use a washcloth with water if needed	Zombies are everywhere
Give a code word	You need to know if he was awake
Keep a record	Success comes in small steps
Don't give up	Training could take three months

Dry Spot Asking some simple questions is a good way to tell if your child is awake enough for my method to work.

So what is our endgame, our goal? I am looking for about two weeks of dry nights in a row. Once you have managed that, your zombie is cured of bedwetting, and you are now a bedwetting slayer. You have done the impossible: you have vanquished the bedwetting zombie from your home, hopefully never to be seen again. Such an accomplishment deserves a reward fit for royalty and will granted to you and your child in the form of a lifetime of dry nights with peaceful, uninterrupted sleep. Congratulations, bedwetting slayer!

4

DAYTIME WETTING PROBLEMS

Basics of Day Wetting

The next most common potty training problem, after bedwetting, is daytime wetting. Children who wet themselves during the daytime are not doing it on purpose. They are usually having these accidents because their brain has not yet gained full control over potty training. If the brain does not provide any control over potty training, a child will have daytime accidents randomly throughout the day. She isn't having these accidents on purpose; it's not her fault. Daytime wetting is a very frustrating potty training problem for parents and children. I hope that you can better understand why this happens after reading this chapter.

Daytime potty problems are common—in fact, we know that the number of children who are having daytime potty problems is increasing. About 7 percent of seven-year-olds have daytime potty problems. These problems decline gradually until about age ten, when only 1 or 2 percent of children still have difficulties with daytime potty problems.

We think that the increasing number of children with daytime potty problems is due to the fact that children are being toilet trained later then they were in the past. We talked about this earlier in this book. When children are trained later, after thirty-two months of age, the risk for daytime potty problems is increased. Even though daytime potty problems are not quite as common as

Figure 3.1   How Common Is Daywetting at Different Ages?

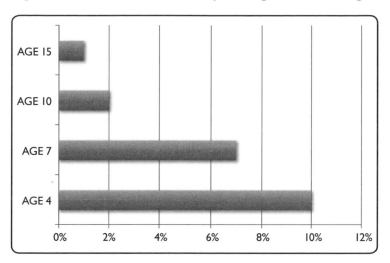

bedwetting, they are much more frustrating for the family and for the child.

Unlike bedwetting, it's hard to keep daytime wetting a secret. Children with daytime potty training problems might wet at school, in the grocery store, or on the soccer field. Because of this, children who wet during the daytime are more likely to be teased and bullied than children who wet the bed at night in the privacy of their homes. Imagine what it must be like for a child to be talking with her friend one minute, and then to have a full-blown accident while standing right in front of her best friend.

Unfortunately, this is a fairly common potty training problem and one that needs to be fixed when it occurs. To deal with day-time potty training problems, children will often go to school with a second set of clothing that they keep handy in the nurse's office. This is not a good situation for the child, and we can help stop these accidents.

We all know that children can sometimes be cruel to each other by teasing and taunting. This would be especially true for children who have urinary accidents during the day. Other children simply don't understand why their classmate might have accidents during the day, and even adults don't quite understand. Unless you are familiar with the information found in this book, you would not know why children have daytime accidents and would probably think it was due to laziness, not caring, or being preoccupied with something else.

I did a study looking at bullying rates in children who wet themselves during the daytime. So far, I have found that children who have daytime accidents tend to have more issues with bullying. This is unfortunate but probably not that surprising. Children who are wet during the day are subject to more bullying and ridicule by their peers than children who don't have problems with urinary leakage during the day. So daytime wetting is a potty training problem that can potentially affect the child's self-esteem.

> **Dry Spot** Children who wet during the day are more likely to be teased than children who only wet at night.

How Common Are Daytime Wetting Problems?

Daytime wetting problems are one of the more common problems that occur after potty training. When I see a child with daytime and nighttime urinary control problems, I always ask the parents and the child, Which problem is worse? If we could make one problem go away, which one would it be? Nine times out of ten, the parent and the child both say that the daytime problem is by far the most bothersome potty training problem that they have. When I hear this, all of our treatment efforts are directed toward trying to reduce or stop the daytime potty problem that the child is experiencing.

School nurses and teachers may also be confused about why children have daytime potty problems. They often think, incorrectly, that the problem occurs because the child is lazy, does not want to stay in class, or is trying to act out. This is not true. The child is not purposely wetting, it is simply a matter of unfinished potty training that could be due to a small bladder, weak stopper muscle, or the fact that the brain has not developed to the point where potty training is even possible.

I had a very nice family come to see me recently because the child was having significant daytime urinary potty problems. She was eight years old and was having accidents at school. She was never able to be completely potty trained. The mother was very concerned and was doing everything that she could to help her child. The child was a very bright little girl who was in the honors program at school. After we evaluated her, we determined that her bladder was normal size, that her stopper muscle was working, but that her brain was still not ready for potty training during the day. The child's urinary leakage problem had absolutely nothing to do with the child's being lazy or spiteful.

However, the school nurse and administration had not read this book and were unaware of these important facts. They assumed that the child was wetting as a signal of a more serious problem like child abuse! The child's parents could not be more caring or attentive to the child, and they were obviously frustrated by the child's potty problem. Because the school did not understand why an eight-year-old child would still have accidents during the day, the school reported the family to the local authorities for evaluation of possible child abuse.

I don't have to tell you that once that charge was made, the authorities had to do a full investigation. The parents went through quite an ordeal and were really in a state of shock about the accusation. Of course, in the end, no evidence of child abuse was found, and we continued to treat the child for daytime potty problems. The child was eventually fully potty trained, and we were able to educate the school system about why children have daytime potty problems.

This is just a dramatic example of how misunderstood daytime urinary control problems can be in children. Daytime potty problems often stem from incomplete potty training during younger ages or from potty training occurring too late. We must remember that the method of potty training doesn't matter, what matters most is that potty training is done at the right time and that it is not delayed. Again, we want to begin to potty train between twenty-seven and thirty-two months of age in order to prevent daytime potty problems later on in life. When daytime potty problems do occur, they can be quite frustrating and can last a very long time. It therefore makes good sense to try to prevent these problems by training at the right time during your child's development.

> **Dry Spot**
>
> Children who begin potty training after thirty-two months of age are more likely to develop daytime potty problems.

Urinary Frequency and Urgency

Not all children with daytime potty problems will leak urine during the day. Some children might just not be able to hold the urine very long. These might be children with small bladders. Even though these children don't wet themselves, the daytime potty problem of going all the time can be very frustrating. Imagine if your child had to go to the bathroom many times each hour.

This problem of urinary frequency and urgency is a fairly common potty training problem. "Frequency" means to go often, while "urgency" means to go suddenly. The typical scenario is that the child is fine one second and then the next second has a severe urge to go to the bathroom. This can be quite frustrating for parents who don't understand how that can happen.

Children with this syndrome may have been previously potty trained and then suddenly start to have episodes where they have to urinate every five or ten minutes. We don't really know what causes the problem, but we think that it might be caused by something irritating the bladder. This irritation could have been something the child ate or was exposed to in the form of an allergen, a laundry detergent, or a fabric softener. We do know that it is nothing to worry about and will usually go away within a few months without any specific treatment. Children with this problem do not have leakage, they just go to the potty all the time.

The typical complaint of parents, and children, who have this problem is that the child has to go to the bathroom much more often than normally. Sometimes children with this syndrome will go to the bathroom every five minutes. Imagine how frustrating that could be. An interesting fact about this problem is that it only occurs during the day. Once the child goes to sleep, the problem goes away for the night but resumes in the morning. Since this problem is thought to be due to bladder irritation or inflammation, we don't consider it a result of incomplete potty training.

> **Dry Spot** Children with the urinary frequency urgency syndrome go potty frequently but do not wet.

Lazy Bladder in Children

Lazy bladder is a potty problem that is usually related to late potty training. Lazy bladder occurs in children who refuse to go potty. Since this can often occur in children who are late to toilet train, it is important to begin toilet training at the appropriate age, between twenty-seven and thirty-two months. Children with lazy bladder will use the potty very infrequently, sometimes only one or two times per day. They hold their urine back because they don't want to go to the bathroom.

Constipation is very common in children with lazy bladder because as they hold back their urine, they also hold back their poop. Children with this problem usually develop urinary leaks because a very full bladder will eventually just have to empty on its own, causing children to have accidents. Eventually, children with this problem can develop urinary tract infections, and, if they hold back their urine too much, the urine has no place to go and will back up, hurting the kidneys.

Of all the potty training problems we discuss in this book, lazy bladder is probably the most important one from a medical standpoint. It is the one potty problem that can hurt your child. You can suspect that your child has this problem if your child uses the potty very infrequently, usually only once or twice each day. Children with this problem also have signs of constipation, such as hard poops or

Figure 4.2   How Lazy Bladder and Constipation Happen

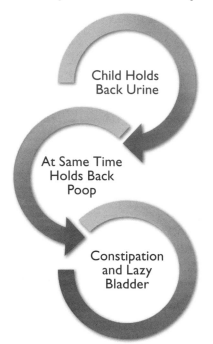

skid marks in the underwear. Once a child develops a urinary tract infection from this problem, parents will usually take her to see the doctor, but you can see your doctor sooner if you think your child has this kind of potty problem.

Treatment for children with lazy bladder includes restarting the potty training process. You have to go back to the basics and start having your child go the bathroom using a watch. Every two or three hours you need to tell your child that it is potty time, even if he doesn't have the feeling to go.

If your child has this problem, it is also important to treat the underlying constipation that develops from constantly holding the urine back. The hard poop pushes against the bladder and can also cause infections. We can treat the constipation by increasing the fiber and water in your child's diet and by making sure that your child poops at least once per day.

Giggle Incontinence

Giggle incontinence is a frustrating problem for children and parents. Parents will often bring their child in to see me because whenever the child laughs hard she will have the complete loss of urine. When I tell them that the name of this condition is giggle incontinence, they start to giggle, and sometimes the child will wet right in front of me.

We are not sure what causes giggle incontinence, but we think it is due to some type of signal that is triggered in the brain whenever the child laughs. This is not a problem that results from incomplete potty training. We think that when the child laughs the brain sends a signal to the bladder that it's time to go to the bathroom, and then the child has an accident.

Giggle incontinence in children is very different from women who develop stress urinary incontinence after childbirth. These women can have episodes of lost urine whenever they run, jump, or laugh. This is due to childbirth's stretching out the muscles that hold the bladder in place. Sometimes parents will bring their children in to see me thinking that their child has stress incontinence, when in actuality they have giggle incontinence.

Giggle incontinence is difficult to treat, but the good news is that most cases will go away with maturity and development. Nothing really needs to be done for giggle incontinence, but if the symptoms are really bothersome there are biofeedback exercises that your child can learn. If you turn to the biofeedback section in chapter 6 of this book you can read about these exercises and how they can help strengthen the stopper muscle to treat giggle incontinence.

Dry Spot Children do not develop stress urinary incontinence, they develop giggle incontinence.

Giggle incontinence also sometimes responds to medications. In the medication section of this book you will learn about anticholinergic medicines. These medications are often very effective for children with giggle incontinence, and they are safe and have few side effects. When these medications are not effective, medications that are used for attention deficit disorder (ADD) can be used, but these medications are more powerful and have more serious side effects. We are not really sure how or why these ADD medications help giggle incontinence, but in some children with severe symptoms they can help.

We have talked about several common daytime potty problems. Children who wet during the day and those with lazy bladder are still not fully potty trained. Children with giggle incontinence or those with urinary frequency and urgency have been successfully potty trained. These problems are not the result of incomplete potty training. So let's focus on children who wet during the day and those with lazy bladder because those are the children who are still not fully potty trained and that is the subject of this book.

Daytime Potty Problems Could Mean Toilet Training Is Incomplete

Children with daytime wetting are really children who have not yet fully toilet trained. But remember that it's not your fault. We know that if your child has not successfully toilet trained it's more likely due to a small bladder, weak stopper muscle, or delay in the brain's ability to potty train. There is not much you can do about those things. So relax and stop feeling guilty that you might have done something wrong during toilet training. You didn't.

So let's focus on what to do now that your child is having ongoing daytime potty problems. Daytime potty problems are not only embarrassing, but they can also lead to urinary tract infections and skin rashes, so it makes a lot of good sense to treat daytime potty problems in children. We don't want to allow these medical problems to occur, and then have to go through unpleasant testing, when everything could be avoided by trying to fix the potty problem from the start.

Now there is nothing we can do to help your child develop faster—other than breastfeeding, and it's too late for that now. Eventually your child will stop having these potty problems during the day, but this could take a long time, and we don't want to just wait around and do nothing. We already said that medical problems could develop and that having potty problems during the day is not really fun. So what else can we do to help our child overcome a daytime potty problem?

How to Stop Daytime Potty Problems in Your Child

The first thing we have to understand is that children who have potty accidents during the day don't have full control over their bladder due to one of three possible reasons that we have already discussed: One, the brain is not mature enough to control the bladder. Two, the bladder might be too small. Or three, the urinary stopper muscle might be weak. So we have to work around these problems if we are to stop the daytime potty accidents from happening.

One big thing we can do is timed voiding or timed urination. This is a very simple skill that you can teach your child that will certainly help with daytime accidents. There is evidence-based information that tells us that timed voiding is an effective way to reduce daytime potty problems in children. Timed voiding is very similar to what we did when we first potty trained your child using a watch. This is how timed voiding works.

> **Dry Spot** Timed voiding takes the responsibility of when to go to the bathroom away from your child.

Pick a time interval such as one hour or two hours, depending upon how often your child has an accident. If your child has an accident every hour, then make the timed voiding interval for your child every hour. If your child only has an accident two or three times per day, make the timed voiding interval two or three hours. When we do timed voiding, we are bypassing the brain and bladder size by reminding your child to go to potty based on time. We do not want to rely on your child to tell us when us when she needs to go to the bathroom. Instead, we want to set up a schedule to bypass your child's sensations. Using this method, we can dramatically decrease the number of accidents that occur during the day.

Timed voiding is not as easy as it sounds, so pay careful attention to the details. Remember that children are playing and having fun, so they don't really have much interest in remembering to go to the bathroom. This is very different than taking a twenty-seven-month-old to the potty on a regular basis. Now we are dealing with an older child who is much more involved with other things. And, unlike when our children were twenty-seven months old, we can no longer watch our children twenty-four hours a day, seven days a week. So we need help to make sure the child goes to the bathroom every two hours even when we are not around to remind them.

A Timed Voiding Strategy That Works

Timed voiding is great for children who don't pay attention when their bladder sends them a signal that it is time to go to the bathroom. I am sure that you have occasionally noticed your child sitting in front of her favorite videogame and wiggling around trying to not urinate so that she could finish the videogame and get an all-time high score. All of a sudden, she can hold it no more and she makes a mad dash to the bathroom and might have an accident along the way. Some children just are too busy with other things to pay attention to their body, and they will do everything in their power to try not to urinate. This is especially true if they are doing something very important like talking to friends or playing on the computer.

Timed voiding is an effective way to overcome your child's preoccupation with other things. It makes potty training front and center of her existence. Here is how it works. First, we pick a reasonable time schedule for your child to go to the bathroom. Even if she has absolutely no desire or interest to go to the bathroom, when that time interval hits, she has to go.

The purpose of starting a timed voiding schedule is to develop consistency for your child, which will reinforce good potty toilet training habits. If we set the schedule for every three hours, then your child has to agree to go to the bathroom every three hours, no matter what. It does not matter if she is watching TV or playing with her friends, if we do a timed voiding schedule, your child has to stop everything and go to the bathroom according to the schedule.

When we use timed voiding, we are taking responsibility away from your child because we recognize that she don't always go when she is supposed to go. We are telling her that we're not going to worry about her body signals for the moment, we are going to instead have her go to the bathroom on a regular schedule, even if she doesn't feel like she has to go to the bathroom. You can tell your child that she can go to the bathroom more often then the schedule, but whenever that three- or four-hour mark hits, she has to agree to go to the bathroom without a fight or fuss.

This will not only develop good potty training habits for your child, but it will also stretch the bladder back to hold more urine if the bladder is small. And as the bladder stretches and your child holds more urine, the stopper muscle will also get stronger. We can therefore see that timed voiding addresses the three possible reasons why your child might still have daytime potty training problems.

There is nothing magical about setting up a time voiding schedule for your child. Just talk to him and have him agree that he will go to the bathroom every three or four hours no matter what. Have him sign a contract if you need to. After that, the difficult part is to make sure that he actually goes every three to four hours during the day. Let's face it, you can monitor your child pretty closely at home, but when he is at school or away at his friend's house, he is basically on his own. We have to let him know how important it is for him to agree to go to the bathroom according to the schedule.

To help your child remember that it is potty time, he can use a wristwatch. There are several different kinds of wristwatches that children can wear to remind them when to go to the bathroom. Of course, there is the standard wristwatch that can beep every three to four hours. I don't like these because they can draw attention to your child, and most children do not want to wear a watch that sounds an alarm every three to four hours. These types of watches are also not practical to use in school, where they can disrupt the entire classroom.

Instead of using a watch that make a noise, your child can use a watch that vibrates. The silent vibration will be a gentle reminder that it is time to go to the potty. These vibrating watches are great for school because they don't make any noise and they don't draw any attention to your child. You can set the watch for any time interval that you want, and the vibration will be the consistent reminder that your child needs to let her know it is potty time. These watches are very successful in helping children remember that it is time to go potty. You can find purchasing information for these vibrating watches in the Additional Resources section of this book.

Dry Spot Using a vibrating watch can be a very effective way to begin a timed voiding program.

Once you have succeeded in using the watch and your child is dry for that time interval, your goal is to gradually increase the time interval. For example, if your child is on a one-hour timed voiding schedule and doing well, the next step should be to increase the interval by thirty-minute increments every three weeks until your child is able to be dry for a three-hour period. This could take several months to accomplish, so be patient and do not expect to see perfect results right away. But if you stick with it, there is no doubt in my mind that your child will eventually become dry during the day.

There are some other important points to consider that will help you succeed. First, let your child know that, when it is time to go potty, she should not rush. Going to the potty is not a race. Once your child actually goes into the bathroom, we have to let her know that it's time to slow down. It's important that she takes enough time to relax and fully empty her bladder. Most children are so busy with other things that they feel they can only spare a few seconds to go to the bathroom. This is not enough time. We have to make sure that your child spends at least three or four minutes in the bathroom to make sure the bladder has enough time to empty completely. There are different timers, like an hourglass filled with sand, that can be used in the bathroom to help your child keep track of time.

So what else can we do? Here is another big thing to consider: constipation has to be avoided. If constipation is present, the poop sits right on top of the bladder, and this reduces the amount of urine that the bladder can hold. Because of this, it is important for you to know if your child is constipated and then treat it if you think it's a problem. It's really not that difficult to determine if your child is constipated, but like anything else you have to look for it in order to find it.

The first thing you need to do is to determine how often your child poops. Most children poop once a day or every other day. If your child is doing that, then at least you know that your child is pooping often enough. Clearly, if your child is only pooping once or twice per week, that is not enough, and you are probably dealing with constipation.

But figuring out how often your child poops is not enough. We also have to know if the poops are soft and well formed like they should be. Or are the poops very large and hard like rocks? In order to figure this out we need to do a poop inspection. After your child poops, you have to look at the poop and inspect it. That's right, you have to be the poop inspector. Take a look at the poop and see if it appears to be of normal size. See if it appears soft and well formed. If it looks like little pebbles coming out of a rabbit or a large poop that came out of a five-ton dinosaur, then your child may be constipated. You should also ask your child if it hurts when she poops because that is a sign of constipation.

If your poop inspection has determined that your child is constipated, you need to fix that in order to help the daytime potty problem. So what can you do? The first thing is to increase the amount of water that your child drinks during the day. Water is the best thing to drink, and if your child is under eight years of age, one additional pint of water per day should be good. If your child is over eight years of age, two additional pints per day should be enough.

In addition to increasing water intake, make sure she is getting enough fiber in her diet. Foods that are rich in fiber should be introduced into your child's diet, and oftentimes this is all that you will need to do. Beans, whole grains, and brown rice are great choices. White rice does not provide much fiber, so be sure to select brown rice. Oatmeal, vegetables, and berries are also excellent sources of fiber that children tend to enjoy. And, for a great snack, popcorn can be offered since it rich in fiber. However, despite all of our best efforts, sometimes it's hard for children to eat enough fiber during the day, so fiber supplements can be helpful.

Dry Spot A poop inspection should include how often your child poops and the size and consistency of the poop.

There are different types of fiber sources that you can use for your child, especially if he doesn't like to eat vegetables and fruits. Fiber supplements are concentrated sources of fiber that work just like other sources of fiber. The way fiber works is this: when you introduce fiber into your child's diet, that fiber is not digested. It's not supposed to be. It passes into your child's colon where it becomes part of your child's poop. Because fiber is dry and soaks up water, it pulls the water that your child drinks into the poop, and when water enters poop, poop becomes softer. That is how fiber prevents constipation. This is why, along with fiber, you want your child to drink lots of water—because, if there is no water around to be pulled into the poop, the fiber can actually make the poops even harder. So make sure your child eats lots of fiber and drinks lots of water, too!

I typically recommend things like fiber chews as fiber supplements, which are available in most supermarkets. Children like to eat sweets, and these fiber supplements taste good, are soft to chew, and are not gritty. You won't usually get into a big fight with your child about eating them, but don't overdo it. One or two fiber chews per day is enough for most children. And remember, have your child drink water with the fiber chew!

Another good source of fiber are fiber cereal bars. These are tasty and will provide enough fiber for almost any child. If your child is under eight years of age, half of a bar should be enough. If your child is over eight years of age, the whole bar should be fine. I also like fiber wafers, one half to one cookie per day. These come in flavors children like and will provide enough fiber to prevent constipation.

There is one important thing you need to remember. When you increase the fiber in your child's diet, it is very important for him to drink plenty of water. Increasing the fiber in your child's diet without increasing water could make constipation worse. This is because the fiber needs liquid in order to be effective. Otherwise, the fiber will be like a pile of dry hay and will make things worse. So, whenever your child eats a fiber supplement, make sure he washes it down with a nice tall glass of water. If he doesn't like water, he can drink whatever fluid he likes. But he must drink that fluid with the fiber.

So now you have placed your child on a timed potty schedule, you are making sure that she takes enough time when she goes to the bathroom, and you are also making sure she is not constipated. You are well on your way to success. These effective techniques will dramatically decrease your child's daytime accidents. Before you know it, your child will be successfully potty trained during the day.

5

MEDICATIONS

Sometimes, despite our efforts, potty training problems just won't go away, and medications are needed. In this chapter, I talk about some of these medications, only those that I personally prescribe and trust. This discussion on medical treatments for potty training is another area that sets this book apart from other potty training books.

There is nothing wrong with using medicine for children with urinary control problems, and it doesn't mean that you have failed potty training. Nothing is 100 percent, and even though we may have tried our best to stop potty training problems, there are still those who need a little extra help. We are very fortunate to have medications available to us that can help.

Most of the medications that I talk about in this chapter require a prescription, so this information is intended for your educational purposes only. If you are interested in starting your child on one of these medications, you certainly need to talk to your doctor.

I have prescribed every one of the medications that I talk about in this chapter. When they're used correctly, they are safe and effective for children with potty training problems. But like anything else, if they are used improperly, they can cause problems. It is important that you use these medications as directed by your physician, and it is important that your doctor be comfortable prescribing these types of medications. Some doctors are not familiar with them.

Some pediatricians would rather have a urologist prescribe medications for potty problems, while others are perfectly comfortable prescribing these medications on their own. This totally depends on your pediatrician, so again you should discuss these possibilities with your doctor and decide upon the best route of action for your child.

There are also situations where you may want to use medication instead of doing some of the things we discussed in this book. Let's say that your child is under a lot of stress and that you don't want to use the bedwetting alarm at a particular time in your child's life. It is perfectly acceptable to use medication instead of the alarm in that situation. You're not doing anything bad by using medication; you can consider medication another option for treating your child.

I often give parents a choice. I describe all of the different treatment options, and then we decide together what the best treatment option for the child is. Oftentimes we start with an approach that does not involve medication, but sometimes medication might be a better choice. For example, if the child has been extremely stressed and depressed about the fact that she is wetting the bed, sometimes a quick fix with a medication will get her motivated to participate in the bedwetting alarm program.

So I don't want you to think that medication is a sign of failure or that it is something that you should avoid at all costs. When used properly, and under the supervision of your physician, medication can sometimes be the best choice for your child. For the remaining part of this chapter we will explore the different medications that are available for children with potty problems, and we will discuss how they fit into the overall treatment programs.

Nighttime Urinary Control Medications

DESMOPRESSIN

The first line of medical approach used for children with bedwetting is desmopressin. This medication works by decreasing the amount of urine that a child makes at night. Parents often tell me that their child makes a tremendous amount of urine at night, soaking first through training pants and then soaking the entire bed. They cannot understand how their small child can make such a significant amount of urine at night. As we discuss desmopressin I think you'll begin to understand why some children with bedwetting actually do make abnormally large amounts of urine at night.

After you go to sleep at night, your body will automatically make a hormone called "anti-diuretic hormone." This hormone is the same thing as desmopressin. When your body makes desmopressin at night, it circulates to the kidneys and tells the kidneys to make smaller amounts of urine because you are sleeping. This hormone is normally released a few hours after you go to sleep at night. So urine production is less at night than it is during the day.

In some children who have bedwetting, this hormone is not released. I think you can imagine what happens. If the kidneys don't get the signal to make less urine at night, and if there is no desmopressin in the bloodstream, then the kidneys begin to make abnormally large amounts of urine. The kidneys just continue to produce urine while your child is sleeping, and this eventually overwhelms the bladder's ability to store it, and bedwetting occurs.

Dry Spot Desmopressin is often considered the first-line medical treatment for bedwetting.

The medication desmopressin is given shortly before bed and restores desmopressin levels to a normal range, which decreases the amount of urine that is made at night. This medication is effective for children who don't produce this hormone at night. Don't worry if your child is not producing the desmopressin on her own. As she matures, she will eventually start to make this hormone on her own. The fact that she is not currently making the hormone is not a indication of an underlying medical problem. It is just part of the developmental delay associated with bedwetting.

The exciting thing about desmopressin is that it works immediately in reducing the amount of urine that is made at night and preventing bedwetting. The medication is given about one hour before bedtime. Because the medication works immediately, it can be used for important events like sleepovers and campouts, or it can be used every day, under the supervision of your physician. But it does not work in all children. It works in about 60–70 percent of the patients who take the medication.

Desmopressin is provided in a nasal spray or tablet form. I have to mention a couple things here: If your physician provides the medication in a nasal spray form, it has to be refrigerated. It is also important that, when your child takes the medication, he doesn't sniff the medication like a typical nose spray. If it is sniffed and then swallowed, this medication will be deactivated in the stomach, and it will not work. If your child is given the nasal spray form of the medication, it should be sprayed into the nose, but your child *should not sniff* during administration. Let the medication be absorbed by the nose.

Desmopressin is also provided in a tablet form. This is more commonly used. The tablet form of the medication is more reliable than the nasal spray, and refrigeration is not required. If your child cannot swallow the tablet with a small sip of water, the tablet can be chewed or placed under the tongue to dissolve. The tablet doesn't have any flavor or taste, so most children who cannot swallow the tablet will happily chew it or let it melt in their mouths.

Both forms of desmopressin should be taken about one hour before the child goes to bed at night to allow sufficient time for the medication to be absorbed into the bloodstream. Another very important fact to remember when using desmopressin is that we want to limit the amount of fluid that the child drinks about two hours before bedtime. This is because desmopressin will prevent the kidneys from making a large amount of urine at night. If the child drinks large amounts of water right before bed, the kidneys will be unable to get rid of this water, and fluid overload can occur. This can lead to headaches, nausea, vomiting, and even seizures, so it is important that your child takes this medication properly and only under the supervision of your doctor. However, this medication is very safe and effective, and I've used it for thousands of children with bedwetting problems.

IMIPRAMINE

The second-line medication for bedwetting is imipramine. This medication belongs to the antidepressant class of medication. It's reserved for children who have not responded to the bedwetting alarm or to desmopressin, typically older children who still have bedwetting problems. Because of the overdose problem associated with this medication, many pediatricians are reluctant to prescribe imipramine and will instead refer patients to a pediatric urologist. This medication has been around for a very long time, and it is prescribed fairly often by pediatric urologists—and it works very well—but, like anything else, it has to be taken properly to avoid side effects and problems.

Overdoses occur when the child takes too much or does not take the medicine as directed. It can result in cardiac arrhythmia problems. So, if your child is prescribed imipramine, it is important that your child take the medication as directed by your physician and not use more than directed.

Dry Spot Imipramine is in the antidepressant class of medication, but it's not used in antidepressant doses for bedwetting.

We are not 100 percent sure how imipramine works for bedwetting. It seems to lighten the sleep stage so the child is a little bit more aware of her bladder filling at night. The sleep stage is not lightened so much that she will wake up tired, just enough to prevent the bladder from emptying at night.

We also think that imipramine works by tightening up the stopper muscle that holds urine inside the bladder. Remember, this muscle must be closed in order for the bladder to hold urine at night. If this muscle is closed, then the bladder can fill and hold more urine. Imipramine also seems to work by allowing the bladder muscle to expand a little bit more at night and hold more urine. So imipramine seems to work in several different ways that, together, make it a very effective medication for bedwetting.

Imipramine is given shortly before bed. It's only available in tablet form, so your child must be able to swallow a pill in order to take it. In my practice, I usually prescribe imipramine for children eleven years of age and older, but it has been used successfully for younger children. The medication is not used in antidepressant doses when it is used for bedwetting, so the antidepressant effects should not be an issue. If you are interested in using this medication for your child, I recommend that you discuss this with your pediatrician in order to determine if this is the right approach. Side effects from this medication can include personality changes or mood swings. Heartbeat problems can result from overdoses.

 Dry Spot Overdose and death from overdose of imipramine has been reported when too much medication has been taken by mistake.

Medications for Daytime Potty Problems

There are all different types of medicine for daytime potty problems in children. Like many medications, most of them have not been fully tested by the Food and Drug Administration (FDA) and are not FDA approved for use in children. This doesn't mean that doctors can't prescribe these medications for children, and it doesn't mean that they aren't safe for children—it just means that they have not been tested or approved for use in children by the FDA.

The reason that these medications have not been tested in children is because it is very expensive to do clinical drug testing and because the market for use of these medications in children is very small. That means that drug companies could spend millions of dollars testing a medication for use in children, but they will never be able to make that money back because the number of children who will actually need this medication is very small. So the drug companies simply don't test the medications in children, and for this reason, there are very few medications that have been approved by the FDA for use in children.

The good news is that recent laws now require all new medications to be tested in children while they are being tested in adults. The government has therefore forced drug companies to perform this testing in children even if they anticipate losing money in the long run because the medications may have a limited market for children. This is a good development for pediatric medicine because it's ideal to test medications in a formal scientific setting before using the medication in children.

The medications that I talk about in this chapter have been used for children for many years; in some cases, the medication has been around for over fifty years. In my opinion, these medications are all safe and effective for use in children who have daytime potty problems. I have prescribed these medications personally in my practice with no significant problems. This does not mean that children can take these medications unsupervised. These are prescription medications, and they need to be provided by your doctor, and all instructions need to be followed very carefully.

ANTI-CHOLINERGIC MEDICATIONS

Anti-cholinergic medications are a group of medicines that calm down the bladder. Remember that, if the brain is not in full control over the bladder, the bladder will empty whenever it wants to. We call this type of bladder contraction an "uninhibited bladder contraction." Side effects for this class of medication include dry mouth, constipation, and temporary facial flushing or redness.

Oxybutynin   There are many different medications in the anti-cholinergic class of medications. The most commonly used medications are oxybutynin, tolterodine, and solifenacin. Let's talk about oxybutynin first since this medication has been around for decades and has proven to be safe and effective in children with daytime potty problems. We generally do not start medication for children with daytime potty problems until the age of four or five, depending upon the child's situation. For example, sometimes a four-year-old can be extremely bothered by a daytime potty problem, especially if it occurs at school. For these children, it may make sense to begin medication therapy if all other forms of treatment have failed.

Oxybutynin acts by calming down the bladder and taking away some of those uninhibited bladder contractions. It just makes the bladder less likely to contract and empty on its own. It's available in a liquid or tablet form and has to be taken two or three times per day in order for it to be effective.

A more modern form of oxybutynin has been developed called oxybutynin XL. This medication only needs to be taken once a day, and the XL stands for the fact that it is a time-release medication. The XL form of oxybutynin has to be swallowed and is available only in pill form. This can be a problem for some children who cannot swallow pills.

Dry Spot Oxybutynin is the least expensive of all anti-cholinergic medications.

Tolterodine and Solifenacin There are other, more modern, medications for children with daytime urinary control issues. These medications include tolterodine and solifenacin and are used by many pediatric urologists to treat daytime wetting problems. These medications work just like oxybutynin but have fewer side effects than the standard form of oxybutynin. They are available only in pill form. These medications are extended-release medications, so they need to be taken only one time per day. This is an advantage for a busy family that is on the go. Sometimes it is very easy to forget to give your child medication. Like oxybutynin, these medications will stop those uninhibited bladder contractions from happening and will reduce the number of accidents that your child is having during the day.

Dry Spot Tolterodine and solifenacin have the advantages of fewer side effects and once-a-day dosing.

Oxybutynin Patch There is also a medication form of oxybutynin that comes in a patch. This is an interesting medication because it is administered by placing a patch on the child's leg or backside. It's an extended-release form of oxybutynin, but since it is in patch form, it doesn't need to be swallowed. This medication is an alternative for children who can't swallow pills and whose parents want the convenience of a once-a-day medication. Like all anti-cholinergic medications, this medication works by relaxing the bladder and preventing unexpected bladder contractions from happening.

All medications in this class have essentially the same side effects and effectiveness. The most common side effects that we see are mild and include dry mouth and some constipation. The newer medications tend to have fewer side effects when compared to oxybutynin. When your child takes these medications, it is important that he drinks lots of water during the day to avoid constipation. As we discussed before, constipation can often be associated with daytime potty problems in children, and we don't want to make that problem worse.

If you are going to start a medication treatment program for your child with a daytime potty problem, it is important that you follow up with your doctor on a regular basis to make sure that the medication is working properly and that there are no side effects. If these medications are taken as directed, they are very effective and safe and provide a way for you to control your child's daytime potty problem.

Dry Spot The oxybutynin patch is an alternative if your child can't swallow a pill.

ALPHA BLOCKERS TAMSULOSIN AND DOXAZOSIN

Alpha blockers are a class of medicines that are occasionally used for children who have daytime potty problems. Some children have problems because their stopper muscle works too much. When these children try to urinate, the stopper muscle makes it difficult for the child to empty the bladder. The child has to push the urine past that tight muscle, and this can result in bladder irritation and child irritability. This condition can also prevent the child from fully emptying the bladder.

Alpha blockers like tamsulosin and doxazosin are being prescribed more often now by pediatric urologists because they are great at relaxing the stopper muscle. These medications are only available in tablet form, and they can sometimes cause some dizziness because they can lower blood pressure, so we usually give this kind of medication right before bedtime.

 Take this type of medication at night before bed to prevent dizziness.

Antibiotics

Antibiotics are not usually used for children with potty problems because urinary control problems in children are not caused by urinary tract infections. Because of this, there is no reason to place a child on antibiotics for toilet training problems.

Sometimes children with potty problems are incorrectly placed on antibiotics because the symptoms that they are having can be confused with a urinary tract infection. For example, some children who develop a urinary tract infection will also start having problems with urinary control. They will suddenly start to have accidents during the day. Typically, these children will also have some other symptoms of a urinary tract infection, like burning with urination or fevers. Because potty training symptoms can be confused with signs of a urinary tract infection, there is a temptation to treat potty problems with antibiotics. This should not be done, and it could lead to antibiotic-resistant bacteria.

Children with urinary tract infections who develop urinary control problems typically have no history of potty training problems. They get an infection and then suddenly will start to have problems with urinary control. This is very different from a child who has always had problems with potty training.

If a child has a potty training problem, she is more likely to develop a urinary tract infection. If she does, her potty training problem usually gets much worse, and she can develop other symptoms, like burning with urination, foul-smelling urine, or low-grade fever. If your child has these symptoms in addition to potty training issues, it is important that you get a urine analysis and culture done by your pediatrician to determine if your child needs antibiotics.

But in general, children with potty training issues do not require antibiotics, and antibiotics should not be used in the hopes of stopping potty issues. When antibiotics are used improperly, like any medication, they can do harm, so they need to be used only when necessary.

> **Dry Spot**   Symptoms of a urinary tract infection can be confused with potty training problems.

ADD MEDICATIONS

ADD (attention deficit disorder) medications are sometimes used for children with giggle incontinence. Some children who leak urine only when they giggle or laugh have been placed on these medications to stop the problem. I generally do not use this class of medicine for this problem because of the side effects these drugs might have. I would rather try to treat this problem with exercises and other medications if the symptoms are very severe.

We are not sure how these medications help children with giggle incontinence. We think that, when a child with giggle incontinence laughs, the laugh triggers some type of signal in the brain for the bladder to empty. We are not sure why some children suddenly develop giggle incontinence, but it can be a very frustrating problem for children. Imagine being at a party with your friends and then suddenly having complete loss of urine because your friend tells a funny joke. This is why the problem can be frustrating, and parents and children often want treatment. For severe cases, ADD medications can be considered as a treatment option, but it needs to be carefully monitored under the supervision of your doctor. Remember, giggle incontinence is not a potty training problem.

ANTI-INFLAMMATORIES

Anti-inflammatories work by reducing inflammation in the bladder. Some conditions, like having to go all the time, are thought to

Table 5.1 Medications Commonly Used for Urinary Control Problems in Children				
Medications	How They Work	Liquid	Tablet	Patch
Oxybutynin	It relaxes the bladder.	Yes	Yes	No
Oxybutynin patch	It relaxes the bladder.	No	No	Yes
Tolterodine	It relaxes the bladder.	No	Yes	No
Solifenacin	It relaxes the bladder.	No	Yes	No
Tamsulosin	It relaxes the stopper muscle.	No	Yes	No
Antibiotics	They kill bacteria.	Yes	Yes	No
ADD medications	They work in the brain.	Yes	Yes	No
Ibuprofen	It reduces inflammation.	Yes	Yes	No

be due to bladder inflammation caused by chemicals that the body releases called prostaglandins. Medications like ibuprofen fight these prostaglandins and stop the inflammation and irritation that they cause. This is why these medications are sometimes used for children who go to the bathroom too much.

Because these medications sometimes work for children who go to often, they have also been used for other children with potty problems like bedwetting and day wetting. The idea is the same, with anti-inflammatories working by reducing the effects of the prostaglandins in the bladder as a way to reduce potty problems. These medications can have side effects like upsetting the tummy or internal bleeding, so even though these are over-the-counter medications, you should only have your child take these for potty training problems if your child is being monitored by your doctor.

6

TESTS AND X-RAYS

If a potty training problem does not resolve or goes on beyond the age of seven or eight years of age, sometimes your doctor might order a test to make sure everything is okay. The good news is that potty training problems are rarely due to any type of medical problem. But, if a potty training problem does not go away after trying all of the things we discussed in this book, it is often a good idea to do some testing. This is especially true if you are thinking about starting medication. In this section we will review all of the tests that your doctor might consider to evaluate a potty training problem.

Urine Analysis

A urine analysis is a very simple test that your pediatrician can do to evaluate your child with a potty training problem. Urinalysis can be done by using a urine dipstick right in the office, and it will provide a very quick assessment of your child's urine. It can tell you things, for example, if there is sugar in the urine, that might suggest diabetes. It also looks for blood and for signs of infection in the urine.

The urine analysis is not necessary for all children who have potty problems, but it is probably a good idea if your child has not responded to treatment or is about to undergo a medication treatment plan under the care of a doctor. If the urine analysis suggests that there might be an infection, a urine culture can be done to see if there is bacteria growing in the urine. Urine culture usually takes forty-eight hours to get results, whereas the urine analysis results are available immediately.

Urine Culture

A urine culture is done when your doctor suspects that your child has a urinary tract infection. A urine culture is not necessary for most children with potty problems. The urine culture looks for bacteria in the urine, and if bacteria is present, then your child has a urinary tract infection. Urinary tract infections need to be treated with antibiotics, since they won't go away on their own. If your child has a urinary tract infection and a potty training problem, then it is important to treat the urinary tract infection first.

 Dry Spot   Ultrasound is a good non-invasive screening test.

Ultrasound

An ultrasound is often done as part of an evaluation when a physician is going to prescribe medication. Ultrasound gives a good overview of the entire urinary tract and does not involve any X-rays. It is not painful or uncomfortable. Because the ultrasound is easy to do and provides a great deal of information, it is a good screening test for many children with potty problems.

Ultrasound will typically look at the bladder and kidneys to determine if they are growing and developing properly. The ultrasound can also look for things like kidney stones and can estimate how big the bladder is.

Biofeedback

Biofeedback is a form of exercise that can be taught to children. This is usually done by a urologist; I don't think there are many pediatricians who teach biofeedback to your child. Biofeedback is done to help the urinary stopper muscle. Basically, little stickers, like electrocardiogram (EKG) patches, are placed onto your child's bottom. The idea is to teach her how to squeeze and strengthen or relax the stopper muscle.

A nurse usually works with your child to teach her how to find these muscles. Once she find the muscles and squeezes them properly, she can then use the stopper muscles to play a videogame as part of the biofeedback exercises.

In this game, when your child squeezes the stopper muscles the electrical impulse created by squeezing the muscle will be transmitted from the EKG patches to a computer game, and the child can do things like shoot asteroids out of the sky or plant flowers. There are variety of different games that your child can play using biofeedback, but the idea is to teach the child to control the stopper muscle.

Uroflow

This is a test that doctors will sometimes do to determine how your child is urinating. It is a very simple test that does not cause any pain or discomfort. Basically your child will urinate into a special container that is connected to a computer. The computer will measure how fast your child urinates and will also measure the action of the stopper muscle to make sure that it's working properly.

 Dry Spot VCUG is not a fun test, but if your child needs it, the test can detect problems to avoid kidney damage.

VCUG

VCUG is a test that is done for children who have urinary tract infections. Since urinary tract infections are more common in children with potty problems, you may run across this term. VCUG stands for "voiding cystourethrogram." Basically, it is an X-ray of your child's bladder while your child urinates. In order to do this test, the radiologist has to put a catheter into your child's bladder through the urethra, which is the tube that your child urinates through. As you can imagine, most children do not like this test at all.

After the catheter is inserted into the bladder, the radiologist will inject contrast (a dye) into the bladder so that the bladder outline can be seen on the x-ray. The bladder will be filled until your child has to urinate. Once your child has to urinate, the radiologist will ask your child to urinate right there on the radiology table. Many children will not want to do this and will fight the urge to urinate. When they fight to urge to urinate, the radiologist will continue to inject more contrast into the bladder until it is impossible for the child to hold any more urine and then the child will urinate. Sounds like a fun test, right?

Many parents will come to me to ask if their child really needs this test after it has been recommended by the pediatrician. Parents will often do anything they can to avoid this test, but if it's done properly, it's not as bad as it sounds. If your child has to have this test, make sure you go to a center that does a lot of these procedures and is comfortable doing them for children. There are also medications that you can give a child before or during this test to make the test more comfortable. Sometimes we can inject lidocaine jelly into the urethra. This is a form of local anesthetic that will make the catheter insertion of little bit easier. Or sometimes we can give the child an oral medication to relax him, something like an oral Valium.

A VCUG is usually done to see if your child has reflux. Reflux is a condition where, when your child urinates, instead of all of the urine coming out through the urethra, some of it goes back up the ureters into the kidneys. This reflux can carry harmful bacteria up into the kidneys and can result in urinary tract infections and, potentially, kidney damage. So when your pediatrician recommends a VCUG, she is really doing so to make sure that your child's kidneys are not in any danger from reflux and urinary tract infections. If your child needs this test, then the best thing to do is to have the test done at a place where they can take care of the special needs of children and do the test as comfortably as possible.

Urodynamics

Urodynamics is a very specialized test that is only done by urologists. This test is done to gain additional information about why your child might have an ongoing toilet training problem. This test is done for children who have tried every type of treatment program that is available, and still yet they still have potty problems. It's often done in combination with a VCUG.

Urodynamic testing is done by inserting a catheter into the bladder through the urethra, just like a VCUG. The test usually will involve taking some X-rays that will give us the exact same information as the VCUG. After the catheter is inserted into the bladder, it's connected to a computer that is specially designed to evaluate potty problems. After the catheter is connected to the computer, the urologist will fill the bladder with contrast, or sometimes just water, and then the computer will analyze what is happening to your child's bladder as the bladder fills. We can determine if your child's bladder sensations are normal, if the bladder is working properly, and if the stopper muscle is working as it should be.

When I see parents in the office, they often want to know exactly why their child is having a potty problem. Urodynamic testing is the test that can tell us precisely what is happening. Without it, we can't say exactly why the child is having a problem, and the best we can do is to provide the best diagnosis we can make based on their symptoms. If your child has gone through all suggested treatment plans and they haven't worked, then we will generally go ahead and do a urodynamic test to get more information about why your child is having ongoing potty problems that are not responsive to any treatments.

7

BONUS EXPERT INTERVIEWS

This is a really special section of the book that I am very proud of. Over the course of my career I have had the very fortunate opportunity to work with some outstanding health professionals. They are experts in their field and can provide further insight and information about toilet training and potty problems. These experts have agreed to allow me to interview them and provide their expertise on the topics I have covered in this book.

You will see that their recommendations are in line with what we went over in the book, but sometimes hearing it in a different way will help you understand things better. The first person I interview is Dr. Dona Schneider. Dona is an assistant dean at the Rutgers School of Public Health. She provides a unique perspective on the history and public health implications of potty training. Dona's husband is a respected pediatrician in Princeton, New Jersey, and this allows Dona to gain additional insight into potty training from the perspective of the pediatrician. Dona and I have worked together on many of the research studies I mention in this book.

Next, I interview Eileen Creenan. Eileen is a registered nurse and is the nursing director for the Pediatric Continence Center at the Bristol-Myers Squibb Children's Hospital at Robert Wood Johnson University Hospital in New Jersey. I think it will be very valuable to hear how Eileen helps children with potty training problems from a nursing point of view. Our Pediatric Continence Center has been open for decades, and we have treated thousands of children. The information that Eileen shares from her perspective as a nurse at the center is slightly different from my perspective as a physician.

Last, I interview Patricia Whitley-Williams, who is the chairperson of pediatrics at Rutgers–Robert Wood Johnson Medical School in New Jersey. Patricia is a pediatrician who has lots of experience treating children with potty training issues, and she has worked with hundreds of pediatricians in her role of chairperson of a large department. She also runs a residency program, so she teaches the next generation of doctors how to be pediatricians. It will be very exciting to hear what she has to say.

These experts clearly have lots of great information to share, and I hope you enjoy these interviews as much as I hope you have enjoyed this book.

Dona Schneider, PhD

Q: *Can you tell us a little bit about your professional background?*

A: I am trained in political science and education, becoming a certified social studies teacher and a reading specialist for K–12. I found that career was not satisfying, so I went back to school to pursue an MA, a PhD, and then an MPH [a master of public health] in epidemiology. I was offered a position at Rutgers examining the pediatric cancer registry in New Jersey and teaching public health. I've been there ever since, primarily teaching epidemiology to both graduate and undergraduate students, pursuing research projects in child and minority health, and now doing a great deal of administration in public health education.

Q: *Can you tell us what evidence-based research means to you and why it's important?*

A: Evidence-based research is the process by which information is developed through carefully designed research information analysis. Results from evidence-based research studies are reviewed by other experts before they are published in scientific journals. Results from evidence-based research can be considered proof rather than opinion because it is the result of sound research.

Q: *What is public health research?*

A: Public health research focuses on the population as a whole or a subset of the population. It identifies differences between groups and seeks to identify risk factors that can be changed to improve the health of populations. It is often said that public health research is preventive in nature, whereas medical research is curative in nature. Both are clearly important, but their purposes differ. Medical research seeks to improve health for individuals with specific diseases or medical problems. Public health research seeks to prevent those diseases or health conditions from occurring in the first place.

Q: *Why is it important for parents to use toilet training information that is backed up by evidence-based research?*

A: Much of the information parents receive about toilet training is just advice, from family and friends, or from popular sources such as paperback books or the Internet. Even information from pediatricians may be strictly opinion—advice given on the basis of what they think works best from their years in clinical practice. Opinions and perceptions are usually based on good intentions, designed to help parents through what might be a difficult process. Unfortunately, opinions and perceptions cannot offer proof that they will actually work. Most important, they may not apply to all situations.

Q: *Why have there been so few studies about toilet training by researchers over the past twenty years or more?*

A: Several popular physicians and psychologists expressed their opinions on parenting, including toilet training, from the mid-twentieth century to the present. Drs. [Benjamin] Spock, [T. Berry] Brazelton, and many others dominated the discussion in the popular media. With so much advice readily available from self-styled experts, who would want to pay for real research on toilet training? Diapers and poop are not sexy research topics, and toilet training has been approached as an individual or family behavioral issue, not a public health issue.

Q: *Is the Internet a good source of toilet training or bedwetting information for parents?*

A: That depends. The general public may not be very savvy at navigating scientific websites. The vast majority of websites are designed to sell something—books, toilet training programs, or other items designed to make their creators money. In addition, those browsing websites may selectively view those sites that support their preconceived ideas about how to proceed with toilet training. It would be a rare parent who would even consider browsing the scientific literature for articles on toilet training research.

Q: *How have toilet training methods used by parents changed over the last twenty years?*

A: Some parents, especially those dependent upon day care centers that will not take children who are still in diapers, remain firmly in the camp of early toilet training over the past twenty years. Many others, however, embraced child-centered toilet-training methods. This may be because the popular media has been flooded with discussions about child development, because other parents in their social circle are following this trend, or because it is easier to wait for child "readiness" than to follow through early with parent-centered training.

Q: *Why do you think children are being toilet trained later now than they were twenty years ago?*

A: Families are busy. In most families, all the adults are working. The popular media tells parents how important it is to wait for children to be "ready" for toilet training, or to show interest.

There is an implication in the popular media that attempting to train too early can leave psychological scars. This turns out not to be true, based on research studies. On the other hand, there is no stigma, or downside, reported in the lay press for parents who opt for later training. However, as we know, the scientific studies do show problems when children are trained late. Most people just do not have access to this information.

Q: *Do you think it is better to toilet train earlier or later in development?*

A: While I am a believer in early training, I recognize that not all parents have the consistency and patience to pull it off, and not every child may be able to succeed at early training. On the other hand, parents watching for their child to show an interest in toilet training will likely have to wait until the resistance of the "terrible twos" wanes. If this resistance goes into the third and even fourth year, toilet training may turn into a long-term parent-child conflict, and toilet training problems can occur.

Q: *Can you tell us why breastfeeding might be important in preventing bedwetting?*

A: There is biologic sense to the theory that the chemical structures in breast milk aid infants in their neurological development. This means that breastfed children may have a developmental advantage for earlier toilet training and perhaps fewer problems with bedwetting.

Q: *Are there any public health problems that can occur from children being toilet trained at a later age?*

A: From a public health point of view, day care facilities with fewer diaper changing stations provide a more sanitary environment for both the workers and the children they care for. Diaper stations mean more chances for cross-contamination, whereas toileting and washing hands are preferable for preventing the spread of infectious diseases.

Q: *Is it possible for parents save money and the environment by train-ing children earlier?*

A: Certainly. Cloth diapers are a onetime cost outlay, but they re-quire laundering and may cause cross-contamination of other laundry if not handled correctly. Disposable diapers are a direct cost to the family budget, and not a small one at that. As dispos-able diapers are not recyclable, they also add to landfill costs.

Eileen Creenan, RN

Q: *What is your professional background?*

A: I am a pediatric nurse with twenty-five years of experience. Since 1996 I have had the unique opportunity to work with Dr. Bar-one to create New Jersey's first, and only, Pediatric Continence Center. I have remained in this role since.

I am a member of the American Nurses Association and the New Jersey State Nurses Association, and I am on the Executive Board of Directors for the Spina Bifida Resource Network of New Jersey.

Q: *Can you tell us about your Pediatric Continence Center?*

A: We are the only center in the state of New Jersey that focuses solely on treating children with urinary control problems. We are also the only hospital in New Jersey that performs a special-ized test called videourodynamics (VUDS) in children. This test combines an X-ray test, to look at the structure of the urinary system, with an urodynamic, or bladder function test, to give Dr. Barone more information about how to formulate an effective treatment plan for the patient with a urinary control issue. If you notice, we call it a Continence Center, not Incontinence Cen-ter. By naming it so, we empower the patient and family, not the problem for which they are seeking treatment.

Q: *What kinds of problems do you treat at the Continence Center?*

A: We treat many problems in our Continence Center. Many children and adolescents have issues with urinary control from different sources. These children can have several diagnoses. An immature, or overactive, bladder is one in which the child feels no sensation to urinate until the last second and then rushes to the bathroom or has an "accident." I am so happy you talked about this condition in this book because it is a very common urinary control problem in children. We also see children with lazy bladder syndrome, another problem described in this book. Children with lazy bladder may not use the bathroom for many hours.

We also see children with constipation. I do want to mention that urinary and bowel issues go hand in hand. These organs are affected by the same nerves and muscles, so generally, if you have a problem with one, you can see a problem with the other. Ignoring one of these systems can worsen the symptoms of the other. At our Continence Center, we screen for bowel and bladder issues in all of our patients and treat both systems with equal importance.

We also see a number of children with urinary control issues due to medical conditions like spina bifida or spinal cord injury after an accident.

Q: *What is the most common problem you treat at the Continence Center?*

A: Immature bladder is our most prevalent problem. This diagnosis is an umbrella including children with frequent or urgent urination, daytime wetting, or a combination of all of these.

I find my biggest role is as educator, consistently "checking in" with a family. By the time the family gets to us, the problem is usually very longstanding, and a great deal of frustration, angst, and even anger or despair play a role in the family's interpretation of the problem. I start by educating them on the nature of the problem; this takes away the guilt from both the parents and the child. You can get the same information that I discuss with my parents by reading this book. Usually, by the end of our first discussion, the family unit seems to be somewhat relieved and encouraged that there is a solution and that they are not alone in this battle. Unfortunately, only approximately 50 percent of families seek treatment for this problem.

We offer both medicinal and non-medicinal approaches to treatment. It is important for our staff to evaluate the family support system before we can recommend a comprehensive treatment plan. Treating these issues is a lifestyle modification, and we all know how difficult it is to follow through on a diet or exercise plan as an adult. For a child, we need full familial and social support to be successful. Education and communication with the children's school nurse and educators on the nature of a student's problem is crucial so that the system can be supportive and sensitive to the child's needs and understand the treatment plan.

Q: *What advice do you give parents who want to begin to toilet training their child?*

A: The best advice that can be given to a parent is to be patient but to start training before thirty-two months of age for the reasons outlined in this book! Oftentimes I see families who claim to have a "toilet trained" child when, rather, they have a toilet trained parent! There is a great deal of societal pressure to train children early. The pressure comes from family members, day care/preschools, and from a level of guilt from within the parent. Just as children grow and mature at different stages, so does their bladder. These children are not lazy, nor is someone a "bad" parent because he cannot toilet train his child. This is where I feel I can be the most effective in advising the family on realistic expectations for their child.

If a child is unable to undress him/herself, acknowledge the need to go, and make the conscious decision to use the bathroom, he/she is not ready. Parents often see the signs of bladder fullness that signal a child may need to urinate—for example, crossing their legs, doing the "pee-pee dance," or fidgeting. That is a good opportunity to encourage the use of the bathroom. I also suggest using a ring that fits into the toilet when training or a potty chair if your child has difficulty sitting on the toilet. Transition from a "potty chair" to a standard-size toilet can be an issue with some children. I find that if children begin on a "big person potty" using a potty ring, they won't be reluctant to switch.

Q: *What do you tell parents when their child finally seems interested in toilet training?*

A: I encourage making the bathroom available; discuss and show the children what it is for. Dress your child in easily removable clothing so that they can get their clothes off quickly if the need arises; overalls, "onesies," and anything with lots of snaps are not good at this time!

It is also important to use consistent language with your child. Whether you prefer the words, pee, poop, urinate, "make," etc., be sure that you, and anyone who cares for your child, are consistent with those same words.

Q: *What method of toilet training do you prefer, the parent or child method?*

A: I prefer the child method, provided it is started before thirty-two months of age. I prefer to call it the "family" method, implying the family is in synch with the child. At the age of toilet training, developmentally, children are asserting their authority and independence. We should be encouraging that, rather than battling that. There will be many battles over other issues. In this method the child has demonstrated a willingness, or want, to use the bathroom, and the parents are supporting that. I can tell you from my own experience I was very in tune to the toilet training experience and had external pressures to "train" my child. However, by making the bathroom available, and allowing it to occur naturally, I was fortunate that my child literally trained himself in a long weekend. Why? Because he was ready!

Q: *At what age do you begin to treat bedwetting at the Pediatric Continence Center?*

A: We prefer not to treat bedwetting until after age six to eight, preferably eight. Developmentally, prior to this age, the child is not ready to tackle this, even if the parents are frustrated. This is where my role is crucial. Education. Parents are frustrated and do not understand the nature of the problem and need a lot of dialogue to understand why this is happening and that it is a common occurrence. Parents need their overwhelming feelings validated. Many parents are ready to be done with the undergarments, extra wash, but usually, the child is unaffected by this and is not ready to begin treatment. Once the child expresses concern or embarrassment related to bedwetting, it is a good time to start treatment, even if the child has not yet reached eight years of age. Sleepovers seem to be a big motivator.

Q: *How do you begin treatment for bedwetting at the Pediatric Continence Center?*

A: We assess that bedwetting is the sole factor first and foremost. When we sit down and interview families, we often see that there are daytime issues as well, even if they are not wetting in large amounts during the day. That initial assessment is what determines the treatment route we take.

Parents often feel that the use of an undergarment (diaper, training pants, etc.) hinders the child in training at night. That is not true. There is no reason for a family to add multiple loads of laundry weekly. If the use of an undergarment is easier and less stressful, by all means, use one! Our treatment programs for bedwetters rarely suggest the removal of the undergarment unless the child and/or family are absolutely against their use.

The family can choose a medicinal route, prescribed by Dr. Barone, and these medicines are described in this book. This is often beneficial because the results are often very quick. The disadvantage to this route is that, with removal of the medication, the problem may resume. They can also choose a non-medicinal approach that incorporates behavior modification and using bio-feedback for retraining of the pelvic (bottom) muscles, which is more labor intensive, but once the problem resolves, it is generally over.

Q: *What tips or advice can you give parents to make any bedwetting treatment program more successful?*

A: It is important to praise the child for effort, not results. Positive reinforcement is always better, both verbally and by actions. A parent can use an age-appropriate reward system for their efforts. Sticker charts work well with younger school-age children. For adolescents, just being dry is often enough reward, but allowing them extra time doing something they enjoy can be a way to reward their efforts.

Q: *Can you tell us your thoughts about the bedwetting alarm and give us any tips you have learned over the years?*

A: The bedwetting alarm is very effective for use with children. It is important to choose an alarm that has a two-step system to shut it off. Some alarms stop making noise if the child wakes just enough to disconnect it. Adding that second step requires more conscious thought. This is the first step toward getting him/her dry. Remember that in the beginning it is a parent alarm. Most children who are bedwetters are very deep sleepers and may not wake to the sound; Dr. Barone calls them "zombies." Like Dr. Barone, I suggest using a different "code word" each night when the parent feels the child is awake. If they remember it the following morning, they were awake. Use of the alarm requires patience. It is not a quick fix, but still a very effective one.

Q: *At what age do you begin treatment for daytime wetting in children at the Pediatric Continence Center?*

A: Children should probably be at least five years old for treatment, depending on severity.

Q: *What advice do you give parents who have children who have day-time wetting problems?*

A: This is often a much more social issue than bedwetting. It is difficult to hide daytime accidents, especially if they are occurring in school. It is important to come up with a plan for when the accidents occur to minimize any social stigma for the child. Many of these children deny being wet. It takes a great deal of understanding to not punish or be upset when they deny or seem unaffected by their accidents.

A parent should also start paying attention to their bowel movements. As stated previously, bowel and bladder go hand in hand. If a child has daytime wetting, he may have a tendency toward constipation.

Q: *Are there any simple things that parents can do to decrease daytime wetting in children?*

A: A parent can do many things to assist their child. Have the child go to the bathroom on a schedule (e.g., every two to three hours) whether they feel the urge to go or not. Don't ask if they have to go, ask them to try to go. If a parent is struggling with getting the child to use the bathroom with reminders, the use of a vibrating watch set for every two hours can take that parent/child struggle away.

When using the bathroom, children should take their time; make sure they are in a relaxed posture. Boys may try sitting. Girls should make sure their underwear is down to their ankles and their legs are apart leaning forward with elbows on knees. Girls can also sit backward on the toilet and lean on the tank.

Children should also be getting enough fluid intake. Water is best. Avoid caffeinated and carbonated beverages as these irritate the bladder and make the child more likely to have an accident.

Ask your child about her bowel movements. Does she go daily? Is it ever hard, or does it hurt when it comes out? What does it look like, very large logs or tiny hard little balls? These questions can lead a parent to determine if the child is constipated, and they can seek treatment for that. Scheduling a regular time every day to sit on the toilet to try to have a bowel movement is good for the child.

Q: *When do you think parents should seek help from their pediatrician if their child has a daytime wetting problem?*

A: A parent should ask their pediatrician whenever they are concerned. If you are not sure, *ask*! There are many causes of daytime wetting, and most are not long term. If a child was dry and suddenly begins to wet, parents should seek their pediatrician's advice because something changed. If the child has never been dry, it is something that should be discussed at each visit. If the pediatrician is not able to assist the family, the doctor will often refer the family to a program such as ours.

Q: *What kind of advanced testing for urinary control problems do you offer at the Pediatric Continence Center?*

A: In the office, we perform uroflow with monitoring of the urinary stopper muscle. This is a test that checks to see how strong the urinary stream is, whether or not there is a blockage or narrowing in the urethra (the tube connecting the bladder to the outside of the body), and if a child's urinary stopper muscle is working with the bladder or against it. After the child urinates, we can use a bladder scanner, an ultrasound device, to see if the child's bladder is empty or not.

In the hospital we perform videourodynamics. This is actually two tests in one. The "video" portion is actually a voiding cystourethrogram (VCUG), which uses X-rays and a dye to see the bladder shape and contour, whether or not the urine backs up to the kidneys, and what everything looks like when the child urinates. So this test looks at the "ingredients" of the urinary system. The second test that goes on at the same time is a urodynamic test. This test looks at bladder function. We are able to see if the bladder is overactive or underactive and if the bladder is holding the amount of urine we would expect. Because both of these tests require a catheter, we do them together to make it easier on the child and allow us to get as much information as possible to develop a successful treatment plan. Most children with urinary control problems do not need this test.

Q: *Do you have any final advice or recommendations for our parents?*

A: We at the Continence Center understand how difficult a urinary control problem can be for a child and family. There are effective treatments out there, but there is no "magic bullet." Each child is unique, and so is his or her treatment plan. Be patient with your child and your health care team, it may take time to find the right solution to your child's problem, but I am sure you will find the right solution for your child. The fact that you have read this book is a sign that you are heading in the right direction.

Patricia Whitley-Williams, MD

Q: *Can you tell us a little about your background?*

A: I am a proud graduate of Simmons College and earned a BS in biology and my MD from Johns Hopkins School of Medicine. I completed my pediatric residency training at Cincinnati Children's Medical Center at the University of Cincinnati and a pediatric infectious disease fellowship at Boston Medical Center at Boston University School of Medicine. I am currently professor of pediatrics and chair of the Department of Pediatrics at Rutgers–Robert Wood Johnson School of Medicine. Throughout my career I have been involved in teaching medical students, residents, fellows, and physicians as well as the general public about the health of children and infections in children. I have practiced medicine for over thirty years. My special areas of interest are pediatric infections such as HIV/AIDS, tuberculosis, and immunizations.

Q: *Toilet training is a major developmental milestone. Where does it fit in with the other developmental milestones?*

A: Toilet training is one of the developmental milestones that is assessed by every pediatrician at age-appropriate visits as part of anticipatory guidance for parents. It is included in the discussion about the child's development in the following four major areas: gross motor (i.e., walking), fine motor (i.e., drinking from a cup), language (i.e., babbling), and social or behavioral skills (i.e., toilet training).

Q: *Do children always reach milestones at the same pace and in the same order?*

A: No, every child develops at his own developmental pace. There is an age range for every developmental milestone during which a child is expected to achieve a certain milestone. Some children might reach that milestone earlier than the expected age, and some later than the expected age. Some children may not achieve the developmental milestones in the same order. An example of this would be a child who has a delayed neurological development in gross motor skills and may not be able to walk independently until two years of age but has achieved the age-appropriate language skills and is able to use two words together by fifteen to eighteen months of age.

Q: *If a child does not reach a developmental milestone when expected, does that mean there is something wrong?*

A: No, pediatricians should reassure parents that each child develops according to his own pace. A developmental assessment should be done by the pediatrician at each visit. This is accomplished by taking a history from the parents as well as observing and examining the child. The pediatrician is trained to recognize a child with developmental delay, and he/she will refer a child as needed for further evaluation by a developmental or behavioral pediatrician. A child will receive early intervention if needed to ensure reaching the maximum potential in achieving every developmental milestone.

Q: *Are there any red flags that parents should look out for if a child does not reach certain developmental milestones?*

A: There are some flags that parents should look out for, including weakness, prolonged tremors, arching of the back, stiffness, failure to follow an object, not making eye contact, not smiling in response to the parent, or failing to turn the head or startle in response to noises. These are just some of the red flags. If there is any concern, especially for first-time parents, the pediatrician should be consulted for evaluation and, in most cases, reassurance.

Q: *There are very few scientific studies on toilet training; why do you think pediatricians have not studied this topic very much?*

A: Much of the data is retrospective, self-reported, and based on questionnaires and surveys. There are so many factors that affect the toilet training of a child that it makes it difficult to control for all of these factors and to conduct randomized, controlled, prospective scientific studies. These factors include, but are not limited to,

- parents' knowledge, skills, attitudes, and beliefs about toilet training,
- the extended family's cultural beliefs,
- the inconsistency in training due to the child being in day care for five out of seven days per week,
- the impact of the use of punishments and/or blame on the child,
- the stressors in the home environment,
- the individual child's neurologic development related to bladder control or ability to pull clothes up or down, and
- the presence of an older sibling in the home to imitate.

Q: *Do most pediatricians receive any kind of formal training or education about toilet training or urinary control problems in children?*

A: In medical school, most of the teaching about toilet training is done during the clinical years in the required third year rotation in pediatrics. This is discussed as part of anticipatory guidance in the ambulatory clinic or private pediatrician's office experience. For a pediatric resident in training, it is presented formally as part of the developmental milestones and anticipatory guidance in the beginning of the internship year and reinforced during direct patient contact in the general pediatric and pediatric urology and/or pediatric nephrology outpatient practices. There needs to be more formal training and education about toilet training or urinary control problems in children.

Q: *What can a pediatrician do to help parents successfully toilet train their child?*

A: Pediatricians should discuss any fears that parents may have about toilet training. The discussion about toilet training should take place as part of anticipatory guidance at successive visits starting at the one-year visit.

Pediatricians should help parents to

- understand that toilet training is a multistep process and a developmental milestone,
- understand that each child will progress at his/her own pace,
- understand that setbacks are common, especially with any stressors in the environment (for example, a move to a new home),
- understand that there is an age range for a child to achieve the goal of being toilet trained,
- help parents to select a method of toilet training that is best suitable for their child,
- offer parents educational materials in print or online to reinforce what was discussed in the pediatrician's office,

* recognize certain behaviors in their child which signal a
  readiness for starting the toilet training process, and
* evaluate the child who has not been able to be toilet
  trained, especially ruling out any gastrointestinal disorders
  (constipation or accidental pooing) or neurologic disorders (such as autism) or identifying conflicting multiple
  caregivers.

Q: *At what age should parents worry if they are unable to toilet train
their child?*

A: Based on a large study involving 1,142 parent questionnaires
from nine pediatric practices in Wisconsin,

* toilet training started at an average age of 27.2 months of
  age and was completed at an average age of 32.5 months,
* girls completed training three months earlier than boys,
* 95 percent of children had a daily or every-other-day bowel
  movement,
* most children aged five to eight years old have regular
  bowel movements, and
* 10 percent were diagnosed as having functional
  constipation.

The most common ages for achieving certain "skills" all or
most of the time:

* Stays bowel movement free overnight—22 months in girls,
  25 months in boys
* "Showing an interest in using the potty"—24 months in
  girls, 26 months in boys
* "Staying dry for two hours"—26 months in girls, 29
  months in boys
* "Indicating a need to go to the bathroom"—26 months in
  girls, 29 months in boys
* Knows how to urinate in the potty—29 months in girls, 31
  months in boys

- Urinates in potty with help—30 months in girls, 32 months in boys
- Uses regular toilet without potty seat—31.4 months in girls, 34 months in boys
- "Staying dry during the day"—32.5 months in girls, 35 months in boys
- Enters bathroom and urinates by self—33 months in girls, 37 months in boys
- "Wakes up dry overnight"—33 months in girls, 36 months in boys
- Enters bathroom and defecates by self—34.4 months in girls, 39.5 months in boys

Is your child ready?

- Does your child enter the bathroom?
- Can your child undress himself/herself?
- Does the child tell you that he/she has to use the bathroom?
- Does your child stay dry at night?
- Does your child sleep through the night without having a bowel movement?

Prepare for toilet training (age eighteen months to four years):

- Discuss with family members.
- Buy a potty seat and leave it in the bathroom.
- Have child observe same-sex older sibling.
- Discuss toilet function to allay any fears the child might have.
- Have a casual, non-punitive, non-coercive, non-blaming approach.
- Give praise when child uses the toilet.
- Do not initiate toilet training at a time of stress in the household.

Q: *Pediatricians are very busy. Should they discuss toilet training problems with their patients?*

A: Yes, pediatricians should always discuss toilet training problems with their patients' parents/caretakers.

Q: *Pediatricians will often tell parents, "Don't worry about bedwetting, your child will outgrow it." While this statement is true, sometimes parents want to treat the bedwetting because the child is getting older or because the bedwetting is bothering the child. What should a parent do in those cases?*

A: The pediatrician should try to reassure them that when the child is developmentally mature enough to sense a full bladder and initiate voiding, he/she will become toilet trained. It is not until four and a half to six years of age that a child can initiate voiding from a full bladder or start and stop the urinary stream at will. The incidence of bed-wetting at three years of age is 40 percent; 30 percent at age four; 20 percent at age five, and 10 percent at age six. Of these, in 15 percent the enuresis [inability to control urination] will resolve. Reportedly, 7 percent of eight-year-olds, 3 percent of twelve-year-olds, and 1 percent of eighteen-year-olds will report bedwetting more than once a month. The latter should have a full evaluation of other causes of enuresis. Twins and parents of children with a history of childhood bedwetting have an increased risk of bedwetting.

The parents can try restricting fluids after a certain hour or after the evening meal as well as having the child urinate at bedtime. Waking up the child at midnight and having the child void sometimes helps as well. The child can practice holding the urine for as long as possible. A reward system could be set up for the child when he/she does not have any bedwetting. Sometimes the technique of imagery has been used to prevent bedwetting. The bedwetting-alarm diaper training method was found to be no more efficacious than the timed-potty diaper method.

There are medications to treat enuresis, but these should only be used in cases in which the bedwetting continues after six years of age and the child has been evaluated for other causes of enuresis. These are associated with treatment failures and relapses. It can take a week or two before any effect is seen. The child should be followed routinely by the pediatrician or urologist.

Q: *What should a parent do if the pediatrician does not want to treat bedwetting, even though the parent and child might want help?*

A: The parent can request from the pediatrician a referral to be seen in a bedwetting clinic or by a pediatric urologist for evaluation and management or a therapist for possible behavioral intervention.

Q: *Is fluid restriction ever a good idea to stop bedwetting or day wetting to children? How much fluid do you think children should drink during the day?*

A: No, the studies on the use of fluid restriction to stop bedwetting have been conflicting. Daily intake of maintenance fluids is 80–100 milliliters (30 milliliters = 1 ounce) per kilogram of body weight.

Q: *Many children with urinary control problems also have constipation. How can a parent determine if their child is constipated?*

A: The definition of constipation in children is a delay or difficulty in defecation for two weeks or more. Infants zero to three months of age should have 2–3 bowel movements per day; six to twelve months of age 1.8 per day; one to three years of age 1.4 per day; and above three years of age 1 per day. I recommend that the child be evaluated by the pediatrician to determine if there is any anatomical or medical reason for the constipation or whether the constipation is behavioral or functional. Most cases of constipation are functional.

Q: *What do you recommend parents do if their child is constipated?*

A: I recommend making sure that the child is getting exercise, drinking fluids, and ingesting adequate fiber such as apples, pears, prunes, raisins, whole wheat bread, beans, grains, etc. (the age plus five = daily intake of fiber in grams). While the studies are conflicting regarding the effect of increased fluid intake on constipation, and the data are not confirmatory on the exact amount of daily fiber needed to prevent constipation in children, adequate hydration and enough fiber in the diet are part of a healthy lifestyle.

Some children may be constipated because of consuming a large amount of dairy. Prior to any restriction in the diet of a child, especially eliminating dairy products, the child should be evaluated by the pediatrician, or nutritionist, and/or a pediatric gastroenterologist.

Dietary changes, medications, especially the chronic use of laxatives, and behavior modification in children should be prescribed and monitored by their pediatrician.

Q: *When do children with constipation need to be seen by the pediatrician?*

A: If they meet the criteria for constipation, they should be seen by their pediatrician. Certainly any child who is complaining of abdominal pain or discomfort from abdominal distension or has blood in the stool should see the pediatrician.

Q: *Do you have any final recommendations or comments for parents?*

A:
   ◆ Be reassured that most children will be toilet trained by age five or six years old.
   ◆ Reward the child when he/she has not had an episode of bedwetting.
   ◆ Regression is common.
   ◆ Remain calm.
   ◆ Refer to your pediatrician and/or a specialist for unsuccessful toilet training.

8

ALTERNATIVE TREATMENTS

Are There Good Alternatives?

So far, we have looked at the standard ways to approach potty training problems and how effective the treatments can be. We also talked about how medications and testing could be used for those troublesome potty training problems that just will not go away. But there are also many alternative treatments, and I would like to discuss these options with you.

I am not opposed outright to any one of these treatments I present here necessarily, but I generally do not use them for my patients because they have not been proven to be effective by scientific studies. In other words, there is no evidence-based information to tell us if these treatments really work.

After reading this book, you can make your own decision. If you think one of these treatments might help your child, you can explore that alternative. But I would encourage you to try the standard treatments before trying one of these alternative treatments. Or at least include a standard treatment along with one of these alternative approaches to potty training problems.

Acupuncture

Acupuncture is an ancient form of Chinese medicine utilizing long thin needles to penetrate the skin to correct imbalances in the flow of energy. It is an Eastern form of medicine that dates back over two thousand years. It probably has benefits if it has survived all of those years. However, we really don't have any evidence-based information that it works or does anything beyond what the acupuncturists claim.

If we look at what the National Institutes of Health say about acupuncture, we learn that they conclude that acupuncture treatment is a type of placebo. This means that the effect of acupuncture may be largely suggestive or psychological. That is, it works because you believe it should work and that you want it to work. It's like taking a sugar pill for pain. But if a child with a potty training problem were to undergo acupuncture, the power of suggestion might not be enough to stop the problem.

If you consider these alternative treatments, it is important to make sure that no harm can come from the treatment. We know that there are scientifically proven solutions that can help, so why should a parent go down this alternative route instead? I believe that parents can sometimes become frustrated if standard treatment does not work and can want to believe that these alternative options will provide a faster solution to their child's potty training problem.

Standard acupuncture treatments for potty training take a long time. If you were to decide to try acupuncture, you should know that most treatment programs last from eight to ten months. You should ask yourself if your child would be willing to undergo these treatments for that many months. Also, do you want to subject your child to a treatment if there is no evidence to show that it works?

All that being said, if you want to give it a try, and if you think your child will respond to this type of treatment, then go for it. Just don't expect miracles, and don't be disappointed if it doesn't work. I have never recommended this treatment for potty training problems. But I have had patients who have come to me after having tried it. As long as it does not traumatize your child, I am okay with giving it a try. You are not being a bad parent if you try acupuncture for your child.

Enemas

We already know that there is evidence that a child who is constipated may also have a potty training issue. We know that constipation can push on the bladder and cause potty problems. We also
know how to gently treat constipation with water and fiber in the
diet. This gentle therapy works for most children with constipation.

But severe constipation causes some children to develop loss of
anal tone, which is caused by stretching of the anus. The child then
has to strain and push for a bowel movement. This occurs because
the stretched-out anal muscle loses power and tone. The lower portion of the bowel, near the rectum, becomes enlarged and dilated,
and it can't effectively push poop out.

When that happens, the solid poop stays in the colon, and the
liquid poop passes around it. It's like a boulder that sits in the colon,
and the only thing that can pass by it is liquid poop. The liquid poop
is pushed around the boulder, and diarrhea comes out. Parents often
wonder how their child could be constipated if he has diarrhea.
Simple: it's because the colon is plugged up by a giant boulder of
poop, so all that gets out is liquid.

So enemas are an alternative therapy that has evidence-based
validity. It is based on things we discussed in this book about constipation and potty training. We know that, as a child becomes constipated and the bowel gets full of poop, the poop exerts pressure
on the bladder, which interferes with potty training and can cause
potty training problems.

In most cases, increasing water and adding fiber to the diet will
treat the constipation. However, if the constipation is severe, something more might be needed, like an enema. I would not start with
enemas, though; I would rather start with something mild like adding water and fiber to the child's diet and go from there. If you are
thinking of using enemas for your child, I would do it under the
supervision of your doctor because enemas can be harmful to children. They can cause rectal tears, and sometimes children can absorb
too much salt and water from the enema fluids. If you treat your child

with enemas, we might also miss finding an underlying medical problem that might be causing severe constipation in your child.

Hypnosis

Hypnotherapy is a natural way to approach your child's potty training problem. Most parents will consider hypnotherapy as a last resort treatment. It is one of the alternative treatments that has not been proven by evidence-based scientific study.

Hypnotherapy is safe, and it makes use of the child's imaginative powers to change her expectations of failure into success. This can be especially helpful for younger children with potty training issues. It leads them into taking control of their body by using imagery and suggestion. These forms of behavior modification can be helpful for some children.

You can also purchase hypnotism CDs instead of going to a hypnotist. Sometimes viewing the CD in the privacy of your home is easier and less scary for your child. Most CDs made for potty training will have the child imagine that she can hold her urine using different forms of imagery.

Because hypnosis uses the power of the child's imagination, it can be effective, especially for children with vivid imaginations. If you work hard at this form of therapy, it can make your child more responsive to more traditional treatments for potty training issues.

Chiropractic

Chiropractic treatment is typically used for adults who have back problems or spine problems. But recent studies have shown that chiropractic might help some children with potty training issues.

A recent study published in the *Journal of Manipulative and Physiological Therapeutics* found that one-quarter of the 171 children in the study treated with chiropractic had a 50 percent reduction in wet nights. That's pretty good success, especially if the children were wet every night before the study began.

It is hard to determine how many treatments might be necessary for children with bedwetting, but you should expect to make three to six visits to the chiropractor before you see improvement. Sessions last about five to ten minutes and can take place two or three times per week. So several weeks are usually needed before you see results. Sometimes results might be seen faster than that, but do not expect to see a change too quickly.

We are not sure how this form of therapy works, but it seems that chiropractic can help the nerves that control the bladder to function better. This could be how chiropractic works for potty training issues, but we are not sure.

9

COMMON QUESTIONS FROM PARENTS

Over the course of the last twenty years, parents have asked me all kinds of questions about toilet training and urinary leakage problems in children. I imagine that I have been asked hundreds of thousands of questions over the years. Although I can't share each question with you—because it would take thousands of pages—I have looked over my extensive experience, and I have summarized it into twenty-five of the most common questions asked by parents.

These questions are here to give you an easy way to get answers quickly without having to look through the entire book. They are the most frequent and important questions that parents have asked me over the last twenty years in my practice as a pediatric urologist, and my answers to these questions will give you the most important and essential information you need. Most of the information found here is explained in more detail in other chapters. But we are all very busy, and sometimes we just need a quick refresher or want information to be at the tips of our fingers.

I hope you will find this chapter to be valuable and informative and that it will provide the kind of beneficial and easily accessible information you need. If any question requires additional information, you can refer to the other chapters or to the index of this book to find a more detailed explanation of the question or topic.

Toilet Training

Q: *How will I know when my child is ready to be potty trained?*

A: Usually you can spot signs of toilet training readiness in your child when he shows some interest in using the toilet. These signs may be subtle, and you may have to look out for them because they could be something as simple as pulling on the diaper or walking toward the potty.

Other signs might include not wanting to spend time in a dirty diaper or wanting to be potty trained just like an older brother or sister. The signs can differ from child to child. If you pay attention to your child's body language, you will be able to spot these signs of toilet training readiness quickly. Nobody knows your child like you do, so I'm sure you're going to be very successful at determining when your child is ready to toilet train.

Q: *Does potty training work best with a potty chair or a real toilet?*

A: I think it is important to use some type of a child-friendly potty to make potty training more successful. One of the most important things that you can do to help your child successfully potty train is to make sure that when she goes to the bathroom everything is nice and comfortable. You want to make sure that the bathroom is warm and that the potty is not too cold or big. You want to make sure that the potty is the right size for your child and that your child's feet can sit comfortably on the floor whenever possible. It's very difficult for children to use the potty if they are struggling to sit on the potty or afraid that they are going to fall in.

There are many inexpensive potty chairs available for you to consider. Some will even play a musical tune when the child goes to the bathroom as a reward. Remember that, when you take your child to his special potty, make a big deal out of it. Tell him how special he is and how proud of him you are that he is using his potty. And once you get him on the potty, make sure you spend enough time with him so he can relax and go. You may need to stop what you're doing, even if it isn't the most convenient time for a potty break.

Getting a good quality potty chair is important, but it is not enough. Time and attention are also important. You have to devote enough time and attention to your child to make potty training successful. This means that you have to spend five or ten minutes in the bathroom to make sure that he is fully relaxed and comfortable and goes to the bathroom. Sometimes reading a favorite book or telling your child a story can help your child relax and will make potty training move along more quickly.

So, I definitely do encourage you to look into getting a good potty chair for your child to make the overall experience of toilet training more comfortable. Some of these potties are portable and can be taken on trips or can be used when you are away from home. Taking a potty with you wherever you go will help you to quickly potty train your child by making sure that potty time is always as safe, comfortable, and familiar as it is at home.

Q: *What toilet training method should I use?*

A: We talked about the two major types of toilet training methods that have been in use over the last hundred years: parent-directed and child-directed methods. Remember that all of the other different types of toilet training are essentially just a slight variation of one of these two forms of potty training.

One form is called the parent-directed method. In this method, the parent initiates the toilet training process and plays a very active role in helping the child toilet train by taking the child to the toilet on a regular schedule and by encouraging the child to use the bathroom on a regular basis. The child-directed approach allows the child to decide when and how to proceed with toilet training. If you use the child-directed method for toilet training, then the parent is more like a facilitator of the toilet training process and acts when the child expresses a desire to go potty.

Our studies have shown that the method of toilet training probably doesn't matter. It is way more important is that you begin toilet training between twenty-seven and thirty-two months of age. You can certainly use the child-directed approach if your child starts to demonstrate signs of readiness toilet train during this age. However, if your child has not demonstrated any signs of total training readiness and is approaching thirty-two months of age, I strongly encourage you to begin toilet training using the parent-directed approach. The method you choose is not as important as making sure that toilet training begins before thirty-two months of age.

Q: *Can I use training pants during potty training?*

A: I think it is perfectly acceptable to use pull-ups both during the day and at night while you are toilet training your child. In my experience, it does not matter much if the child is going to use training pants or underwear during the potty training process. What is more important is that you stick with a dedicated approach to potty training and don't waver once you begin.

I think it is perfectly acceptable to use training pants while potty training your child, but don't use them as an excuse to not take your child to the toilet. For example, let's suppose that you are very busy doing some work on your computer and that your child is playing quietly in training pants. All of a sudden, your child states he has to go to the bathroom, right at the moment when you about to respond to an important e-mail from someone at work. Would you be less likely to take your child to the bathroom knowing that he is in training pants? As long as you answered No! to that question, then it is okay to use training pants during potty training.

Sometimes we might think that it's okay to let a child go in the training pants "just this once," but that could really ruin weeks of toilet training efforts and confuse the child. We have to be consistent with our children when we are training, so if we are going to use training pants, we have to use them with the intent that they are not going to be used as a convenience for us when potty time comes at an inconvenient time or place.

Q: *How long does it take to potty train?*

A: Once you begin potty training, it is a learning process, and like anything else that a child has to learn, it takes time. You don't learn how to do addition or subtraction overnight, and you don't learn how to control your bladder overnight, either. We have to be patient and let our children learn how to control their bladders at their own pace. In general, most children will take two to four months to gain daytime urinary control. This means that, if you begin toilet training by twenty-seven months, your child will probably be trained during the day by thirty-two months of age, given the normal variation of how successful children are when they train. Once your child is dry during the day and doing well without having any accidents, the ability to control urine at night comes a bit more slowly. So, let's not rush things or be too unrealistic when looking at nighttime urinary control. Nighttime urinary control will usually follow daytime urinary control by at least six months. Sometimes nighttime control could take another year or two before your child is dry at night.

Now if you have truly been dedicated and have been trying to toilet train your child for twelve months and have not gotten anywhere, then I want you to go back and read the chapter in this book about potty training and make sure that you are following all the steps properly. Make sure you're not missing anything because even a small variation from what you need to do might influence whether or not you're successful. If you go back and read the chapter again, and you have done everything as instructed, then I recommend that you take a break. Forget training for a little while.

Take the focus completely off potty training and go back to using training pants or a diaper for a month. That's right, completely forget about trying to potty train your child for a month. Sometimes we all just need a break when things are not going right to recharge our batteries. By taking a short break from potty training activities we can usually start fresh, and that is often helpful.

If you are unsuccessful after another four months of training efforts, I suggest that you consider discussing the difficulties that you are having with your pediatrician. The reasons that children might not successfully train, such as constipation, are examined in this book.

Q: *What should I do if my child does not want to toilet train?*

A: It's not uncommon for some children to not be interested in toilet training. Sometimes children are perfectly comfortable staying in dirty diapers and don't show an interest in toilet training. They might even think that toilet training is a strange thing to do when staying in a diaper is perfectly logical to them.

And let's face it, some children are stubborn and simply like resisting anything that you might suggest. This stubbornness is often seen when children start developing a sense of independence, and it usually occurs when children reach about thirty to thirty-six months of age. This is why it is important that you not delay training beyond thirty-two months of age. You need to take charge and begin toilet training if your child is approaching thirty-two months of age and is still is not interested in toilet training.

Q: *I have tried everything to potty train my child and nothing seems to work. What else can I do?*

A: The first thing I would like you to do is to go back and read the chapters in this book that apply to potty training. You might also want to read about how your child gains urinary control during the day. This might give you a better understanding of why you are having difficulties. Pay careful attention to all of the details in the book and follow my advice step-by-step.

Also make sure that there is no chance that your child might be constipated, so read the section on constipation. Remember that constipation can make potty training more difficult because the constipation presses on the bladder and makes the bladder capacity smaller than it actually is.

If you have been trying to potty train for a while, take a break for a few weeks and start again. Use the parent-directed method,

where you take your child to the bathroom during the day while
he is awake. To start, take your child every hour and then, each
week, increase the time interval until your child can last three
hours between potty breaks without having an accident during
the daytime.

Q: *My child will only use the potty at home. Is there anything I can I
do when we are out?*

A: Yes, you can use a portable child potty. It's not uncommon that
children will only want to use a potty that they are comfortable
with. If this sounds like your child, then just go with the flow,
don't try to fight it too much. There are many different potties
that you can use when you're traveling. This is not a forever situation, but right now your child wants the comfort of using her
own potty, just like you might like using your own tennis racket
when you play tennis. If that is what your child wants, and that
is what it takes to get her to successfully toilet trained, then just
let her have her way.

When you think about it, it's not really a big deal; eventually
your child will learn how to use other potties and won't be so
particular. As your child becomes trained, you can slowly introduce different toilets as your child becomes more comfortable.
But right now, our main goal is to get your child toilet trained.
If that means that you need to bring a potty with you wherever
you go, then that's just the way it is for the time being. There is
nothing wrong with a child wanting to use his own potty, and
trust me, someday your child will use other potties. How many
adults have you seen lugging around their own potty, after all?

If your child seems fixated on using one particular potty, it's
not the end of the world, and it doesn't mean that something is
terribly wrong with your child. It just means that your child has
grown very fond of his particular potty. He will probably be very
successful at potty training, but you may need to be a little bit
flexible and simply let him use his potty.

Q: *How long do I let my child sit on the potty each time in an attempt to go?*

A: I think in most cases, if you allow five to ten minutes for each potty break, that is a reasonable amount of time. Make that time productive, and follow all the instructions outlined in this book, such as making sure that the potty is warm and comfortable, that the surroundings are inviting, and that you have a book or story ready to share with your child during potty training breaks. Once your child is comfortable, relaxed, and sitting on the potty, then I would give her five to ten minutes to complete her business before you move on.

Stay focused on the task at hand—even if you are at a baseball game and it's the ninth inning, tie game, bases loaded, bottom of the ninth. It does not really matter where you are or what you're doing, you have to allow five to ten minutes to let your child complete his business. Once that time has passed, if your child still has not gone potty, then remove him from the potty and try again at the next voiding interval. Just be on the lookout for signs of having to go to the bathroom before the next voiding interval if your child was not able to go during the regularly scheduled time.

This is a good question because one of the most difficult things to do is to not be rushed during potty training. Sometimes thirty seconds can seem like thirty minutes when things are busy. It can therefore be helpful if you actually use a watch to time each potty break because waiting with your child for him to go to the bathroom could distort your perception of time, and it is important that you have a realistic idea of how much time you are actually spending in the bathroom. You can use the timer on your phone, or you can buy small hourglass timers filled with sand that you can flip over. These are nice because they can be used to time toilet training, and they will also give your child a visual idea of how much time they have to go to the bathroom. These types of small potty training aids are available at many different stores and outlets. More information can be found in the resource section of this book.

Q: *Should I consider my child potty trained even though the occasional daytime accidents still occurs?*

A: I think you probably should consider your child completely potty trained even if, on occasion, he still has an accident. Nobody is 100 percent perfect after learning a new task or skill, so I would not become terribly upset if your child has an occasional accident during the day. This is probably due to not paying attention to his own body signals when he may be busy doing something else that he considers to be more important than potty time. Just be patient with him; slip-ups and mistakes can happen, but they should resolve with time and encouragement.

However, having an occasional accident is different from having many accidents during the day. Many accidents that occur during the day on a regular basis could be a sign of daytime control issues. These kinds of problems are more often associated with underlying constipation or result from starting the toilet training process after thirty-two months of age. If your child seems to be having multiple accidents during the day on a regular basis, then read the chapter in this book that deals with daytime urinary control problems for advice and more insight into why your child might be having so many accidents during the day.

Daytime Wetting

Q: *My child wets during the day. Is he doing this on purpose?*

A: When your child is having daytime urinary control problems, it is usually because of a combination of several factors. The most common factor is that your child is not paying attention to his body signals and that he is having accidents because he is not going to the bathroom when he is supposed to. When this happens, it is very important to make sure that your child is going to the bathroom on a regular basis. A simple way to do this is with timed voiding. You might remember that timed voiding means that you take your child to the bathroom at a regular time interval whether or not your child wants to go to the bathroom. This is a very helpful technique for children who don't pay attention to their body signals and have accidents because they are not paying attention. So one of the first things that I ask a parent to do if their child is having frequent daytime urinary control issues is to get him on a schedule where he goes to the bathroom every hour or every two hours regardless of whether or not he wants to go to the bathroom.

This can be a struggle sometimes because a child with daytime urine or control problems either doesn't want to go to the bathroom or doesn't have proper signals coming from her bladder to the brain telling her that it is time to go. When you establish a schedule for her, this takes all of the responsibility away from the child and places it on your shoulders. If you are able to successfully use this scheduled approach to toilet training and your child is still having accidents in between the times when you take her to the bathroom, then it could be that other problems are contributing to the daytime urinary control problem.

One of the most common problems that causes a child to have these accidents during the day is constipation. Remember, if the constipation presses on the bladder, then the bladder does not have the ability to fill, and it becomes irritable, so accidents are more common. If you think your child is constipated, then you have to treat the constipation by increasing water and fiber in the diet. Good sources of fiber are whole grains, berries, and oatmeal, and don't forget popcorn for that special treat. You could possibly use a dietary fiber supplement if your child won't eat foods that are rich in fiber. Again, you might want to read the section in this book about constipation if you think your child is having problems with constipation. You can tell if your child is constipated if the stools are hard, or if your child complains of pain when he goes to the bathroom, or if your child has a bowel movement less frequently than every other day.

If you have placed your child on a schedule to go to the bathroom every hour or two, and if there is no chance that your child has constipation, then you may be dealing with a daytime urinary control problem. At this point I suggest you go back and read the daytime wetting chapter in this book because it is important for you to understand why your child is having these daytime accidents. It is important for you to understand that your child is not having these accidents because she is lazy or because she likes to sit and wet her underwear. If you read the chapter, you will soon realize that your child's bladder is simply misbehaving; it is acting independently of the child and is causing the child to have these accidents through no fault of her own. It is terribly important that you understand why children are having these accidents so that you don't resort to any type of punishment or yelling to try to make the daytime urinary control problem better. If you resort to these measures, I can almost guarantee that the problem will get worse.

Q: *Why does my child wait until the last minute to go to the bathroom and then have an accident?*

A: It may look like your child is waiting to the last minute, but in actuality your child is just getting a late signal from the bladder. When you have to go to the bathroom you gradually sense the urge that your bladder is filling and that it will soon be time to go to the bathroom. You might have a sense that you could last anywhere from fifteen minutes to a half an hour before your bladder is ready to really go and you can't hold it anymore. We all have been in a car or on a train and have had the urge to go, but we are able to hold it until we get to a bathroom because the urge to go builds gradually; it does not come on all of a sudden.

Now imagine if your bladder isn't working properly and doesn't warn you that you'll need to empty it soon. Let's say that you feel perfectly fine one second and that the next second your bladder feels like it is ready to explode. You've had no warning; you've had no signal that your bladder was getting full; all of a sudden you just feel like you have to go or else. This is basically what happens to children who appear like they are waiting until the last minute to go to the bathroom.

They have no warning signal because their bladder is not working properly. The signal between the brain and the bladder is not traveling up and down the tracks like it should, so the brain does not have the ability to send a warning signal. The bladder may just declare, "I am ready to go," and if the child can't go to the bathroom immediately, an accident will occur. To the outside observer, this looks like the child was waiting until the last second to go. In reality, the child responded immediately as soon as the bladder gave the signal that it was ready to go. The problem was there was no warning signal for the child.

We have to be aware that children who appear to wait to the last minute to go are probably suffering from an overactive bladder. If you go back and read the daytime wetting chapter in this book, you will get a better understanding for why children develop these problems. For our purposes, it's important to recognize that the child did not wait until the last minute to go—he responded as quickly as possible. The problem was that he didn't get a warning signal from the bladder.

Q: *My child has daytime wetting and constipation. Is this common?*

A: This is very common. When children have daytime urinary control problems they often try to hold back their urine from coming out of the bladder. They do this by tightening up the muscle that prevent urination. We learned that this muscle is called the "external sphincter muscle" in an earlier chapter. It's the stopper muscle. When the child holds this muscle tightly, she not only stops urination but causes constipation because she is also tightening up the muscles that release poop. Constipation develops along with daytime wetting. The more she tries to avoid daytime wetting, the worse the constipation gets. So this becomes a vicious cycle that needs to be broken. We need to teach children how to relax those muscles so that constipation does not develop.

Another reason for constipation in children with daytime urinary control problems is that they believe that limiting fluid intake will stop their urination. But we learned that limiting fluid is never a good idea and that children will still have daytime urinary control problems even if they limit their fluid intake. Remember that daytime urinary accidents have nothing to do with the amount of urine in the bladder; it happens because the bladder empties on its own whenever it wants to and is not under complete control of the brain.

When a child does not drink enough water during the day, the urinary control problems will still continue—and the child will also start to develop constipation. If the child does not drink enough fluid, his poop will become hard and dry, and this will lead to constipation and even pain during pooping. As the constipation worsens, so, too, will teach urinary control problems.

Make sure that your child is pooping once a day or once every other day and that the poop is soft and well formed. If you don't see this, then your child is possibly constipated, and we need to help by increasing fluid and fiber in the diet. Constipation and daytime urinary control problems go hand-in-hand, and it is important to be on the lookout for these kinds of problems.

Q: *Does my child have a medical problem because he has a urinary control problem?*

A: No, your child does not have a medical problem just because he has a urinary control problem. Most children with urinary control problems that occur during the day or at night have immature development of the part of the nervous system that is involved with bladder control. If the bladder is not under control of the brain, then the bladder will empty whenever it wants to. This is similar to a baby's bladder, where the baby will urinate multiple times during the day wherever she is. This is why when children have urinary control problems we sometimes will say that these accidents are due to immature bladder function.

As your child's nervous system matures, most of these urinary control problems will resolve on their own. This is why many pediatricians say that no treatment is necessary because your child will naturally outgrow the problem over time. However, outgrowing bedwetting and daytime wetting problems can be very slow, and sometimes it is better to treat the problem rather than to put up with accidents for years and years.

Q: *My child's urine smells. Does this mean he has an infection?*

A: Bad-smelling urine is not usually a sign of urinary tract infection, although, whenever a child does get a urinary tract infection, the urine can be smelly. It is more common that children have smelly urine without being infected. Some of the most common reasons that children have bad-smelling urine are that they do not drink enough water, or it might have to do with the kind of food that ate, or they do not urinate often enough.

If children don't drink enough water during the day, the urine can be very concentrated and acidic. The concentrated urine, like anything else that is concentrated, will have a stronger odor than less-concentrated urine. When you concentrate any liquid, the smell coming from that liquid is stronger—this is the difference between a perfume and cologne; perfume is more concentrated than cologne and has a stronger smell. Likewise, if your child does not drink enough water during the day, the urine is more concentrated and will have a strong smell. But this doesn't mean your child has an infection. It simply means that your child needs to drink more water during the day.

Food can also influence the smell of a child's urine. There are certain vegetables—like asparagus—that can give urine bad smell. Too much red meat in the diet can also cause foul-smelling urine. Most strong spices like garlic and onions can do the same. So before rushing your child off to the pediatrician for a urine analysis and culture, try to remember what your child ate the night before and see if any of those foods could be contributing to the bad-smelling urine.

Another reason that children's urine might smell is if they don't urinate often enough. Some children will hold their urine for a long time during the day. When the urine sits in the bladder for a long period of time, different chemicals in the urine break down and release substances that produce a strong order. It's like the difference between a pond and a running stream. When water runs in a stream, there is very little odor coming from that stream. But if the water stays still, like it does when it sits in a pond on a hot summer day, the different bacteria and substances in that water can produce an odor. The same is true for the bladder. If your child is urinating on a regular basis, then the bladder is functioning more like a stream, then the urine will not smell. If your child holds his urine all day, than the bladder acts more like a pond, and the urine will break down and release substances that cause a terrible smell.

So, to summarize, if your child is having problems with smelly urine, make sure she is drinking enough water for the urine to be clear or light yellow in color. Remember what your child ate the night before to see if any foods might be causing the smelly urine. Just remember that strong-smelling foods can produce smelly urine. Finally, make sure that your child is urinating on a regular basis every three or four hours during the day and not holding it for six to twelve hours each time between urination. If you follow these simple steps, your child will have a clear urine without bad smells or odors.

Q: *What can I do about a rash that always occurs because my child is constantly wet?*

A: Most rashes that occur in children with daytime or nighttime urinary control problems are caused by substances in the urine breaking down the protective layer of the skin. This can lead to redness, itching, fungal infection, and even abrasions and bleeding. It is important to make sure that your child's skin remains healthy, as it protects against infection.

The best thing to do to prevent skin rashes and breakdowns

is to use a barrier cream with zinc oxide or one of the diaper rash creams that are available at most stores. These creams act as a barrier and prevent the urine from coming in contact with the skin, which prevents skin rash. The idea is to try to prevent the rash from starting in the first place.

Sometimes, despite using these barrier creams, a rash will develop anyway because of the amount of wetness that the child has. Once a rash is established, then a barrier cream is no longer effective, and something else must done. In these cases, an over-the-counter cream with hydrocortisone is often effective. Antifungal creams are also very good because most of these rashes are caused by fungus growing in the child's warm wet area. There are also combination creams that use hydrocortisone and an antifungal, and these can also be very effective.

If the rash is severe and does not respond to over-the-counter medications, you might want to see your pediatrician for a stronger cream. You don't want the rash to get so severe that it starts to cause bleeding and infections.

Bedwetting

Q: *My child is dry during the day but occasionally wets at night. Is my child lazy?*

A: Of course not. It is not uncommon for children to occasionally wet the bed at night even though they arc completely potty trained during the day. Children will usually gain daytime urinary control three to six months before they obtain nighttime urinary control. It's not unusual that every now and then a child might have an occasional accident at night. It does not mean that potty training has been unsuccessful or that your child is lazy. It simply means that your child's potty training process in terms of development is not yet fully complete. There is nothing to worry about, and with a little more time and patience, these occasional nighttime accidents will go away.

Q: *Why does my child wet the bed?*

A: Children wet the bed for many different reasons, so it is not possible to know exactly why your child wets the bed. In most cases
it's due to more than one particular reason. First, let's look at
hereditary factors. If you or your spouse was a bed wetter, then
your child has a 40–80 percent chance of wetting the bed. This
is a very common reason that some children wet the bed. But if
you were a bed wetter and wet the bed until a certain age, it does
not mean that your child will also wet the bed until that age.

Another reason that children wet the bed is that they are very
deep sleepers. When they sleep very deeply, sometimes the signal
from the bladder to the brain does not get through, and the brain
does not have the ability to turn off the bladder at night. When
the brain has no control over the bladder, the bladder will empty
at night without the brain's permission. This is a very common
reason that many children wet the bed, and it is due to the immaturity of your child's nervous system. It does not mean that there
is anything wrong from a medical standpoint, it just means that
your child's nervous system has not matured to the point where
nighttime urinary control as possible. As your child grows and
develops, the nervous system will mature, and nighttime urinary
control will happen.

Sometimes children sleep so deeply that they also snore. This
can be a sign of something called "obstructive sleep apnea." This
is a condition that can be diagnosed only with a special kind of
study called a "sleep study." Children who have sleep apnea need
a sleep study to determine if they are breathing normally during
sleep. If sleep apnea is detected, it needs to be treated for bedwetting to improve. This is because obstructed breathing causes the
release of a hormone that causes the body to make large amounts
of urine at night, and this increases the risk for bedwetting. Signs
of sleep apnea include snoring during sleep and should also be
suspected if your child is overweight.

In some children, excess urine production at night can also
happen if they don't make a hormone called "anti-diuretic hormone." This hormone is normally produced after a child goes to

sleep at night. Without this hormone, your child's kidneys will continue to make large amounts of urine while he is sleeping, and this could overwhelm his bladder's capacity to hold urine all night. Even though some children do not make enough of this hormone at night, we don't consider it to be a medical problem or issue. It's a developmental delay, and with time, your child will eventually start to make this hormone. There is a medication called "desmopressin" that is given to some children with bedwetting problems; it restores hormone levels to normal levels and stops bedwetting in up to 60 percent of children who take this medication.

Q: *Do I have to worry that a medical problem might be causing my child's bedwetting?*

A: Bedwetting is never considered to be a medical problem. If your child wets the bed, you don't need to worry that an underlying medical condition is causing it. Even if bedwetting continues in an older child, we don't consider it to be caused by a medical issue. Many parents often ask me when I would consider bedwetting to be a medical problem, and the answer to that question is "never." I am not saying that bedwetting is not a problem in that it is not bothersome. I'm just saying that, even if it occurs in a sixteen-year-old, an underlying medical problem is not the cause of the bedwetting.

Q: *I had a bedwetting problem until age fifteen. Will my child have the same problem until the same age?*

A: No, there is no relationship between when a parent's bedwetting stopped and when her child's bedwetting might stop. The only thing that we know is that, if you or your spouse had a bedwetting problem, then your child is more likely to have a bedwetting problem. There are actually some genes for bedwetting that have been located on chromosome numbers 8, 12, and 13, and we believe that this is how bedwetting is passed down from parent to child. But those genes can act in different ways in your child than they did in you. You might have wet until you were twelve or thirteen years of age, but that does not mean that your child will do the same. It is completely possible that your child might stop bedwetting at seven or eight years of age. There is really no way to predict. The only thing we can say is that, if you wet the bed, your child has a 40 percent chance of wetting the bed, and if both you and your spouse wet the bed, then your child has an 80 percent chance of wetting the bed. Those are pretty amazing percentages, and it just shows how important hereditary factors are for bedwetting.

Q: *Is it possible that my child might not outgrow bedwetting?*

A: I hate to say this, but there is a small possibility that your child will never outgrow bedwetting. It's a small risk of probably 1 percent, but this is still something that you need to be aware of. Because not all children will outgrow bedwetting, I think it's important to address bedwetting early and treat it like a medical problem even though it is not due to a medical condition. I do see children in my practice who are approaching college age, and the fear starts to set in when parents don't know what their child is going to do when living in a dorm at college.

If you address bedwetting early and develop a good treatment program for your child that is based on the information in this book, I think you will be successful in stopping bedwetting. I also believe that it is easier to treat a bed wetter when she is younger than when she is older, so my advice would be to treat bedwetting early. If your child does not spontaneously stop wetting the bed by age six, then I think that would be a good time to begin a bed-wetting treatment program, which would probably include using one of the bedwetting alarm systems discussed in this book.

Q: *My child is somewhat overweight. Can this contribute to his bed-wetting?*

A: We did a research study that found that being overweight by itself does not increase the risk for bedwetting. In our study, there was no increased risk for bedwetting in children who were overweight. However, in children who are overweight, there is an increased risk of developing obstructive sleep apnea. This is a condition that causes interruption of breathing during sleep. When this occurs, the body will react by making more urine than it is supposed to. This increased urine production will sometimes cause bedwetting. Our study found that children who were overweight and who also had sleep apnea were more likely to wet the bed.

So you should worry about sleep apnea if your child is overweight and also snores loudly at night. Sleep apnea can not only cause bedwetting but also cause behavioral and learning problems at school, so it is an important condition to diagnose and treat. If your child does not snore at night, it is unlikely that your child has sleep apnea.

Q: *Can medication cause my child to wet the bed?*

A: There are not really any medications that are associated with bedwetting. Over the last twenty years I have seen thousands of children with bedwetting, and many of them have been on all different kinds of medications. But I have never seen any medication cause bedwetting. However, if your child never wet the bed but suddenly started to have bedwetting problems after he started taking a certain medication, then it would be reasonable to stop that medication if possible and see if the bedwetting goes away. But in general there is no association between any particular medication and bedwetting.

Q: *What can I do to help my child stop bedwetting?*

A: You're doing it right now by reading this book. Just by being interested in your child's bedwetting, by wanting to play an active role in stopping it, you have gone a long way in helping your child overcome this problem. I encourage you to read this entire book in addition to this chapter, which is meant to be a brief overview of some of the important questions that parents ask. I think that, the more you know about bedwetting and the more you know about your child's urinary system, the better. You will be able to help your child stop bedwetting.

If bedwetting is bothering your child, I think that's a good time to treat the bedwetting. But you don't have to simply wait for your child to want to address the problem because outgrowing bedwetting could take many years. And remember, there are treatments that we can use that could potentially stop bedwetting in as little as two months, so let's get started and face bedwetting head-on and stop it.

Q: *Does disciplining/punishing help with bedwetting?*

A: There is no place for punishment in any bedwetting treatment program. Remember that your child is not bedwetting on purpose or doing it because she is trying to be bad or is acting out. Your child is having this problem because of a developmental delay that is not under her control. It makes no sense at all to punish your child for something she has no control over. In fact, punishing a child for bedwetting could make things even worse by making the child revert to an earlier stage of development in terms of how she reacts to others and copes with the overall problem of bedwetting.

Rewards are a different story. Rewards can help motivate the child to be involved in the bedwetting treatment program. This is especially important if you are using an alarm system. When you use an alarm system, the child has to be willing to wear the alarm every night and be motivated to use it. Sometimes a reward system using stickers or stars on a chart can be a good motivational factor that you can use to keep your child interested in the bedwetting treatment program. So punishment is not ever a good idea, and rewards are always appropriate.

CONCLUSIONS

I hope you have enjoyed our journey to successful toilet training and dry days and nights for your child. One of the main goals of this book has been to present information that is evidence based. This means that the information that we count on in this book is based on scientific studies and not just on someone's opinion or recommendation. It is backed by fact, and it is the best information that is available right now for your child.

We certainly covered a lot of information that for me represents a lifetime of work and study. I hope I have conveyed some of this information to you in an understandable and meaningful way that can help you better understand your child's urinary control problem or help you better understand the best method for potty training your child. Whatever your particular need or interest might be, I hope that I have helped you in at least a small way.

We started out by talking about how children used to be potty trained very early, as early as eighteen months, but then how over the years the average age of potty training has increased to nearly three years of age. We talked about how this delay in potty training age has been associated with an increased incidence of toilet training problems like daytime wetting, and we talked about how important it is to begin potty training between twenty-seven and thirty-two months of age.

The different toilet training methods we discussed include the child-directed method, where the child controls the total training process. We talked about why I prefer the parent-directed toilet training method—because it allows the parent to begin the toilet training process at the proper time. We also talked about some unusual methods of toilet training, like infant toilet training.

I hope you now know how constipation can affect the urinary system and urinary control. It's important to recognize that, if your child is constipated, you can take common steps to treat it by increasing water and fiber in your child's diet. Remember that your child should poop once a day or at least once every other day. The poops should not be hard, and pooping should not be painful for your child.

You probably now have a better understanding of the urinary system then many medical students! You understand the kidneys, and what they do, and how they make urine. You also know that the ureters are the tubes that carry the urine from the kidneys to the bladder. You understand that the bladder is a storage container for urine and that there is a muscle called the "urinary sphincter muscle"—the stopper muscle—that keeps the urine in the bladder. Finally, you know that the entire urinary system is under the control of the brain and that this brain control is critically important for urinary control.

Because of the brain's control, the bladder is able to hold urine and to not have accidents at inconvenient times. If the brain is not in full control of the bladder, then accidents will occur both during the day and at night. But you now know that this is not caused by any medical problems; it's just due to developmental delay of the nervous system. As your child grows and matures, eventually this control will occur, and the urinary control problems will stop. But you also know that the maturation process can take a very long time, so sometimes it is better to treat these problems than to wait years and years for the problems to go away. And that is where this book comes in.

This book gives parents an opportunity to learn about the different toilet training methods and what to do when things go wrong. It teaches parents how to address problems like daytime wetting and nighttime wetting, two very common problems that children can experience during growth and development. I really want to make sure that parents understand that, if their child does have a daytime or nighttime urinary control problem, they do not have to wait for their child to outgrow it. Help and treatment are available.

I also talked about some of the medications that can be used for these problems, along with alternative treatments like chiropractic. These are less-established treatments for bedwetting, but they have been used successfully in children, and I think it's reasonable to keep an open mind about them.

I would like to thank you for taking the time to explore this book with me, and I wish you the best of luck in your journey to successful toilet training, dry nights, and dry days.

GLOSSARY

BIOFEEDBACK This is a treatment that uses an external signal like a video game to help children learn how to control muscles like the urinary sphincter muscle (the stopper muscle for the bladder).

BLADDER The organ that stores and empties urine

CHILD-DIRECTED METHOD OF TOILET TRAINING A toilet training method where the parent waits for the child to be ready to train

CONSTIPATION Hard or infrequent bowel movements

CONTINENCE Being dry and not having any accidents or urine leakage

DESMOPRESSIN This is the hormone the body makes to decrease the amount of urine made at night, and it is available as a medication.

DOXAZOSIN A medication that relaxes the urinary sphincter muscles, used sometimes for children with lazy bladder

ENURESIS Another term for wetting. Day enuresis is wetting during the day, and night enuresis (or nocturnal enuresis) is bedwetting.

EVIDENCE-BASED INFORMATION Information that is backed up by research

FREQUENCY Urinating often, more than once every hour

IMIPRAMINE A medication that is used for bedwetting, particularly in older children

INCONTINENCE Wetting or having a urinary accident during the day or at night

KIDNEYS The organs that make urine

OXYBUTYNIN A medication used for day wetting

PARENT-DIRECTED METHOD OF TOILET TRAINING A method of toilet training where the parent begins and directs the process

SOLIFENACIN A medication that is used for children with day wetting

TAMSULOSIN A medication that relaxes the urinary sphincter muscles, used sometimes for children with lazy bladder

TIMED VOIDING Urinating by using a schedule rather than by relying on body signals

TOILET TRAINING READINESS Signs that suggest that a child is ready to toilet train, like a child not wanting to be in a dirty diaper

TOLTERODINE A medication used for day wetting

URETERS The tubes that carry urine from the kidneys to the bladder

URGENCY The need to urinate suddenly and without warning

URODYNAMICS A special test that can help determine why a child is having a urinary control problem

VCUG A test that is often done if a child has a urinary tract infection

ZOMBIE A child who is really, really hard to wake up

ADDITIONAL RESOURCES

Books for Children

Accidental Lily by Sally Warner (New York: Knopf, 2000).

The Candy Corn Contest by Patricia Giff (Topeka, KS: Econo-Clad Books, 1999).

David's Secret Soccer Goals by Caroline Levine (Philadelphia: Jessica Kingsley Publishers, 2004).

Do Little Mermaids Wet Their Beds? by Jeanne Willis (Morton Grove, IL: Albert Whitman, 2004).

Dry Days, Wet Nights by Maribeth Boelts; illustrated by Kathy Parkinson (Morton Grove, IL: Albert Whitman, 1994).

Prince Bravery and Grace: Attack of the Wet Knights by Gail Ann Gross (Ashton, MD: Brookville Media, 2007).

Waking Up Dry: A Guide to Help Children Overcome Bedwetting by Howard Bennett (Elk Grove Village, IL: American Academy of Pediatrics, 2005).

Books for Adults

The Complete Bedwetting Book: Including a Daytime Program for Nighttime Dryness by D. Preston Smith, MD (Knoxville, TN: PottyMD, 2006).

Getting to Dry: How to Help Your Child Overcome Bedwetting by Max Maizels (Boston: Harvard Common Press, 1997).

Seven Steps to Nighttime Dryness: A Practical Guide for Parents of Children with Bedwetting by Renee Mercer (Ashton, MD: Brookeville Media, 2004).

Waking Up Dry: A Guide to Help Children Overcome Bedwetting by Howard Bennett (Elk Grove Village, IL: American Academy of Pediatrics, 2005).

Other Resources

American Academy of Pediatrics
www.aap.org

Bristol-Myers Squibb Children's Hospital
at Robert Wood Johnson University Hospital
http://bmsch.org

International Children's Continence Society
www.i-c-c-s.org

MedlinePlus: Toilet Training and Bedwetting
(National Library of Medicine)
www.nlm.nih.gov/medlineplus/toilettrainingandbedwetting.html

National Association for Continence
www.nafc.org

National Kidney Foundation
www.kidney.org/patients/bw/

Rutgers–Robert Wood Johnson Medical School,
Division of Urology
www.rwjurology.com

Society for Pediatric Urology
www.spuonline.org

Bedwetting Alarm Manufacturers

Nite Train'r Alarm
Koregon Enterprises, 9735 S.W. Sunshine Court, Suite 100,
   Beaverton, OR 97005, or call 800-544-4240.

Nytone Alarm
Nytone Medical Products, 2424 South 900 West,
   Salt Lake City, UT 84119, or call 801-973-4090.

Night Hawk
www.nighthawkbedwetting.com

Wet-Stop Alarm
www.wetstop.com

Online Resources for Bedwetting Alarms, Vibrating Watches, Books, and Other Supplies

The Bedwetting Store
www.bedwettingstore.com

Potty seats and chairs recommended by *Parents* magazine
www.parents.com/toddlers-preschoolers/potty-training/gear/
best-potty-training-toilets

INDEX